Virtual Clinical Excursions—General Hospital

for

deWit:
Fundamental Concepts and Skills for Nursing,
2nd Edition

Virtual Clinical Excursions—General Hospital

for

deWit:
Fundamental Concepts and Skills for Nursing,
2nd Edition

prepared by

Susan C. deWit, MSN, RN, CNS, PHN
Formerly, Instructor of Nursing
El Centro College
Dallas, Texas

software developed by

Wolfsong Informatics, LLC
Tucson, Arizona

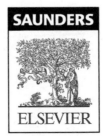

SAUNDERS

ELSEVIER

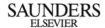

11830 Westline Industrial Dr.
St. Louis, Missouri 63146

Notice

Knowledge and best practice in this field are constantly changing. As new research and experience
broaden our knowledge, changes in practice, treatment and drug therapy may become necessary or
appropriate. Readers are advised to check the most current information provided (i) on procedures
featured or (ii) by the manufacturer of each product to be administered, to verify the recommended
dose or formula, the method and duration of administration, and contraindications. It is the
responsibility of the practitioner, relying on their own experience and knowledge of the patient, to
make diagnoses, to determine dosages and the best treatment for each individual patient, and to
take all appropriate safety precautions. To the fullest extent of the law, neither the Publisher nor
the Authors assumes any liability for any injury and/or damage to persons or property arising out
or related to any use of the material contained in this book.

ISBN 13: 978-1-4160-3034-8
ISBN 1-4160-3034-4

Executive Editor, Nursing: *Tom Wilhelm*
Managing Editor: *Jeff Downing*
Associate Developmental Editor: *Jennifer Anderson*
Project Manager: *Joy Moore*

Printed in the United States of America

Last digit is the print number: 9 8 7 6 5 4

Workbook
prepared by

Susan C. deWit, MSN, RN, CNS, PHN
Formerly, Instructor of Nursing
El Centro College
Dallas, Texas

Textbook

Susan C. deWit, MSN, RN, CNS, PHN
Formerly, Instructor of Nursing
El Centro College
Dallas, Texas

Introduction

This workbook has been constructed to enhance theory learning, but it is specifically directed at helping the student transfer knowledge to the clinical area. After completing the activities in this Virtual Clinical Excursion, students find they are more comfortable entering the hospital. For some activities in this workbook, students are asked to consult a pharmacology book, drug handbook, or medical-surgical text, just as they must when preparing for a clinical assignment or caring for a patient. When there is a need to verify information from their textbook, *Fundamental Concepts and Skills for Nursing*, 2nd edition, the relevant page numbers are given.

Contents

Table of Contents
deWit:
Fundamental Concepts and Skills for Nursing, 2nd Edition

Unit Seven: Medication Administration

Unit Eight: Care of the Surgical and Immobile Patient

Unit Nine: Caring for the Elderly

Getting Started

GETTING SET UP

■ MINIMUM SYSTEM REQUIREMENTS

WINDOWS™

Windows Vista®, XP, 2000 (Recommend Windows XP/2000)
Pentium® III processor (or equivalent) @ 600 MHz (Recommend 800 MHz or better)
256 MB of RAM (Recommend 1 GB or more for Windows Vista®)
800 x 600 screen size (Recommend 1024 x 768)
Thousands of colors
12x CD-ROM drive
Soundblaster 16 soundcard compatibility
Stereo speakers or headphones

Note: Virtual Clinical Excursions—General Hospital for Windows will require a minimal amount of disk space to install icons and required dll files for Windows 98/ME. Windows Vista® and XP require administrator privileges for installation.

MACINTOSH®

MAC OS X (10.2 or higher)
Apple Power PC G3 @ 500 MHz or better
128 MB of RAM (Recommend 256 MB or more)
800 x 600 screen size (Recommend 1024 x 768)
Thousands of colors
12x CD-ROM drive
Stereo speakers or headphones

■ INSTALLATION INSTRUCTIONS

WINDOWS™

1. Insert the *Virtual Clinical Excursions—General Hospital* CD-ROM.
2. The setup screen should appear automatically if the current product is not already installed. Windows Vista users may be asked to authorize additional security prompts.
3. Follow the onscreen instructions during the setup process.

   If the setup screen does *not* appear automatically (and *Virtual Clinical Excursions—General Hospital* has not been installed already):
      a. Click the **My Computer** icon on your desktop or in your Start menu.
      b. Double-click on your CD-ROM drive.
      c. If installation does not start at this point:
         (1) Click the **Start** icon on the taskbar and select the **Run** option.
         (2) Type d:\setup.exe (where "d:\" is your CD-ROM drive) and press **OK**.
         (3) Follow the onscreen instructions for installation.

MACINTOSH®

1. Insert the *Virtual Clinical Excursions—General Hospital* CD in the CD-ROM drive. The disk icon will appear on your desktop.

2. Double-click on the disk icon.

3. Double-click on the GENERAL-HOSPITAL_MAC run file.

Note: Virtual Clinical Excursions—General Hospital for Macintosh does not have an installation setup and can only be run directly from the CD.

■ HOW TO USE VIRTUAL CLINICAL EXCURSIONS—GENERAL HOSPITAL

WINDOWS™

1. Double-click on the *Virtual Clinical Excursions—General Hospital* icon located on your desktop.
2. Or navigate to the program via the Windows Start menu.

Note: Windows 98/ME will require you to restart your computer before running the *Virtual Clinical Excursions—General Hospital* program. If your computer uses Windows Vista, right-click on the desktop shortcut and choose Properties. In the Compatability Mode, check the box for "Run as Administrator." Below is a screen capture to show what this looks like.

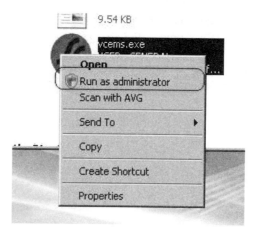

MACINTOSH®

1. Insert the *Virtual Clinical Excursions—General Hospital* CD in the CD-ROM drive. The disk icon will appear on your desktop.

2. Double-click on the disk icon.

3. Double-click on the GENERAL-HOSPITAL_MAC run file.

■ SCREEN SETTINGS

For best results, your computer monitor resolution should be set at a minimum of 800 x 600. The number of colors displayed should be set to "thousands or higher" (High Color or 16 bit) or "millions of colors" (True Color or 24 bit).

Windows™

1. From the **Start** menu, select **Control Panel** (on some systems, you will first go to **Settings**, then to **Control Panel**).
2. Double-click on the **Display** icon.
3. Click on the **Settings** tab.
4. Under **Screen resolution** use the slider bar to select **800 by 600 pixels**.
5. Access the **Colors** drop-down menu by clicking on the down arrow.
6. Select **High Color (16 bit)** or **True Color (24 bit)**.
7. Click on **OK**.
8. You may be asked to verify the setting changes. Click **Yes**.
9. You may be asked to restart your computer to accept the changes. Click **Yes**.

Macintosh®

1. Select the **Monitors** control panel.
2. Select **800 x 600** (or similar) from the **Resolution** area.
3. Select **Thousands** or **Millions** from the **Color Depth** area.

■ WEB BROWSERS

Supported web browsers include Microsoft Internet Explorer (IE) version 6.0 or higher, Netscape version 7.1 or higher, and Mozilla Firefox version 1.4 or higher.

If you use America Online (AOL) for web access, you will need AOL version 4.0 or higher and one of the browsers listed above. Do not use earlier versions of AOL with earlier versions of IE, because you will have difficulty accessing many features.

For best results with AOL:
- Connect to the Internet using AOL version 4.0 or higher.
- Open a private chat within AOL (this allows the AOL client to remain open, without asking whether you wish to disconnect while minimized).
- Minimize AOL.
- Launch a recommended browser.

■ TECHNICAL SUPPORT

Technical support for this product is available between 7:30 a.m. and 7 p.m. (CST), Monday through Friday. Before calling, be sure that your computer meets the minimum system requirements to run this software. Inside the United States and Canada, call 1-800-692-9010. Outside North America, call 314-872-8370. You may also fax your questions to 314-523-4932 or contact Technical Support through e-mail: technical.support@elsevier.com.

Trademarks: Windows, Macintosh, Pentium, and America Online are registered trademarks.

Copyright © 2006 by Elsevier, Inc.

ACCESSING *Virtual Clinical Excursions—General-Hospital* FROM EVOLVE ─────────────

The product you have purchased is part of the Evolve family of online courses and learning resources. Please read the following information thoroughly to get started.

To access your instructor's course on Evolve:

Your instructor will provide you with the username and password needed to access this specific course on the Evolve Learning System. Once you have received this information, please follow these instructions:

1. Go to the Evolve student page (http://evolve.elsevier.com/student)

2. Enter your username and password in the **Login to My Evolve** area and click the **Login** button.

3. You will be taken to your personalized **My Evolve** page, where the course will be listed in the **My Courses** module.

TECHNICAL REQUIREMENTS

To use an Evolve course, you will need access to a computer that is connected to the Internet and equipped with web browser software that supports frames. For optimal performance, it is recommended that you have speakers and use a high-speed Internet connection. However, slower dial-up modems (56 K minimum) are acceptable.

Whichever browser you use, the browser preferences must be set to enable cookies and JavaScript and the cache must be set to reload every time.

Enable Cookies

Browser	Steps
Internet Explorer (IE) 6.0 or higher	1. Select **Tools → Internet Options**. 2. Select **Privacy** tab. 3. Use the slider (slide down) to **Accept All Cookies**. 4. Click **OK**. -OR- 3. Click the **Advanced** button. 4. Click the check box next to **Override Automatic Cookie Handling**. 5. Click the **Accept** radio buttons under **First-party Cookies** and **Third-party Cookies**. 6. Click **OK**.
Netscape 7.1 or higher	1. Select **Edit → Preferences**. 2. Select **Privacy & Security**. 3. Select **Cookies**. 4. Select **Enable All Cookies**.
Mozilla Firefox 1.4 or higher	1. Select **Tools → Options**. 2. Select the **Privacy** icon. 3. Click to expand Cookies. 4. Select **Allow sites to set cookies**. 5. Click **OK**.

Enable JavaScript

Browser	Steps
Internet Explorer (IE) 6.0 or higher	1. Select **Tools → Internet Options**. 2. Select **Security** tab. 3. Under **Security level for this zone** set to **Medium** or lower.
Netscape 7.1 or higher	1. Select **Edit → Preferences**. 2. Select **Advanced**. 3. Select **Scripts & Plugins**. 4. Make sure the **Navigator** box is checked to **Enable JavaScript**. 5. Click **OK**.
Mozilla Firefox 1.4 or higher	1. Select **Tools → Options**. 2. Select the **Content** icon. 3. Select **Enable JavaScript**. 4. Click **OK**.

Set Cache to Always Reload a Page

Browser	Steps
Internet Explorer (IE) 6.0 or higher	1. Select **Tools → Internet Options**. 2. Select **General** tab. 3. Go to the **Temporary Internet Files** and click the **Settings** button. 4. Select the radio button for **Every visit to the page** and click **OK** when complete.
Netscape 7.1 or higher	1. Select **Edit → Preferences**. 2. Select **Advanced**. 3. Select **Cache**. 4. Select the **Every time I view the page** radio button. 5. Click **OK**.
Mozilla Firefox 1.4 or higher	1. Select **Tools → Options**. 2. Select the **Privacy** icon. 3. Click to expand Cache. 4. Set the value to "**0**" in the **Use up to: __ MB of disk space for the cache** field. 5. Click **OK**.

Plug-Ins

Adobe Acrobat Reader—With the free Acrobat Reader software, you can view and print Adobe PDF files. Many Evolve products offer student and instructor manuals, checklists, and more in this format!

Download at: http://www.adobe.com

Apple QuickTime—Install this to hear word pronunciations, heart and lung sounds, and many other helpful audio clips within Evolve Online Courses!

Download at: http://www.apple.com

Adobe Flash Player—This player will enhance your viewing of many Evolve web pages, as well as educational short-form to long-form animation within the Evolve Learning System!

Download at: http://www.adobe.com

Adobe Shockwave Player—Shockwave is best for viewing the many interactive learning activities within Evolve Online Courses!

Download at: http://www.adobe.com

Microsoft Word Viewer—With this viewer Microsoft Word users can share documents with those who don't have Word, and users without Word can open and view Word documents. Many Evolve products have testbank, student and instructor manuals, and other documents available for downloading and viewing on your own computer!

Download at: http://www.microsoft.com

Microsoft PowerPoint Viewer—View PowerPoint 97, 2000, and 2002 presentations even if you don't have PowerPoint with this viewer. Many Evolve products have slides available for downloading and viewing on your own computer!

Download at: http://www.microsoft.com

SUPPORT INFORMATION

Live support is available to customers in the United States and Canada from 7:30 a.m. to 7 p.m. (CST), Monday through Friday by calling **1-800-401-9962**. You can also send an email to evolve-support@elsevier.com.

There is also **24/7 support information** available on the Evolve website (http://evolve.elsevier.com), including:

- Guided Tours
- Tutorials
- Frequently Asked Questions (FAQs)
- Online Copies of Course User Guides
- And much more!

A QUICK TOUR

Welcome to *Virtual Clinical Excursions—General Hospital*, a virtual hospital setting in which you can work with multiple complex patient simulations and also learn to access and evaluate the information resources that are essential for high-quality patient care. The virtual hospital, Pacific View Regional Hospital, has realistic architecture and access to patient rooms, a Nurses' Station, and a Medication Room.

■ BEFORE YOU START

Make sure you have your textbook nearby when you use the *Virtual Clinical Excursions— General Hospital* CD. You will want to consult topic areas in your textbook frequently while working with the CD and using this workbook.

■ HOW TO SIGN IN

- Enter your name on the Student Nurse identification badge.
- Next, specify the floor on which you will work. The Medical-Surgical Floor is automatically chosen next to **Select Floor**. If you wish to select another floor (Skilled Nursing or Obstetrics), click the down arrow to access the menu. For this quick tour, choose the Medical-Surgical Floor.
- Now click the down arrow next to **Select Period of Care**. This drop-down menu gives you four periods of care from which to choose. In Periods of Care 1 through 3, you can actively engage in patient assessment, entry of data in the electronic patient record (EPR), and medication administration. Period of Care 4 presents the day in review. Highlight and click the appropriate period of care. (For this quick tour, choose **Period of Care 1**.) Click **Go**. This takes you to the Patient List screen (see example on page 11). Only the patients on the floor you choose (Medical-Surgical) are available. Note that the virtual time is provided in the box at the lower left corner of the screen (0730, since we chose Period of Care 1).

Note: If you choose to work during Period of Care 4: 1900-2000, the Patient List screen is skipped since you are not able to visit patients or administer medications during the shift. Instead, you are taken directly to the Nurses' Station, where the records of all the patients on the floor are available for your review.

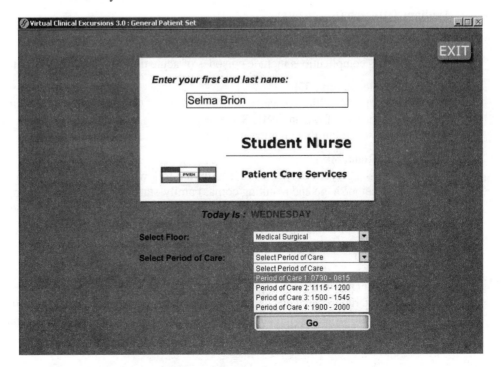

■ PATIENT LIST

MEDICAL-SURGICAL UNIT

Harry George (Room 401)
Osteomyelitis—A 54-year-old Caucasian male admitted from a homeless shelter with an infected leg. He has complications of type 2 diabetes mellitus, alcohol abuse, nicotine addiction, poor pain control, and complex psychosocial issues.

Jacquline Catanazaro (Room 402)
Asthma—A 45-year-old Caucasian female admitted with an acute asthma exacerbation and suspected pneumonia. She has complications of chronic schizophrenia, noncompliance with medication therapy, obesity, and herniated disc.

Piya Jordan (Room 403)
Bowel obstruction—A 68-year-old Asian female admitted with a colon mass and suspected adenocarcinoma. She undergoes a right hemicolectomy. This patient's complications include atrial fibrillation, hypokalemia, and symptoms of meperidine toxicity.

Clarence Hughes (Room 404)
Degenerative joint disease—A 73-year-old African-American male admitted for a left total knee replacement. His preparations for discharge are complicated by the development of a pulmonary embolus and the need for ongoing intravenous therapy.

Pablo Rodriguez (Room 405)
Metastatic lung carcinoma—A 71-year-old Hispanic male admitted with symptoms of dehydration and malnutrition. He has chronic pain secondary to multiple subcutaneous skin nodules and psychosocial concerns related to family issues with his approaching death.

Patricia Newman (Room 406)
Pneumonia—A 61-year-old Caucasian female admitted with worsening pulmonary function and an acute respiratory infection. Her chronic emphysema is complicated by heavy smoking, hypertension, and malnutrition. She needs access to community resources such as a smoking cessation program and meal assistance.

SKILLED NURSING UNIT

William Jefferson (Room 501)
Alzheimer's disease—A 75-year-old African-American male admitted for stabilization of type 2 diabetes and hypertension following a recent acute care admission for a urinary tract infection and sepsis. His complications include episodes of acute delirium and a history of osteoarthritis.

Kathryn Doyle (Room 503)
Rehabilitation post left hip replacement—A 79-year-old Caucasian female admitted following a complicated recovery from an ORIF. She is experiencing symptoms of malnutrition and depression due to unstable family dynamics, placing her at risk for elder abuse.

Goro Oishi (Room 505)
Hospice care—A 66-year-old Asian male admitted following an acute care admission for an intracerebral hemorrhage and resulting coma. Family-staff interactions provide opportunities to explore death and dying issues related to conflict about advanced life support and cultural and religious differences.

OBSTETRICS UNIT

Dorothy Grant (Room 201)
30-week intrauterine pregnancy—A 25-year-old multipara admitted with abdominal trauma following a domestic violence incident. Her complications include preterm labor and extensive social issues such as acquiring safe housing for her family upon discharge.

■ HOW TO SELECT A PATIENT

- You can choose one or more patients to work with from the Patient List by checking the box to the left of the patient name(s). For this quick tour, select Piya Jordan. (In order to receive a scorecard for a patient, the patient must be selected before proceeding to the Nurses' Station.)
- Click on **Get Report** to the right of the medical records number (MRN) to view a summary of the patient's care during the 12-hour period before your arrival on the unit.
- After reviewing the report, click on **Go to Nurses' Station** in the right lower corner to begin your care. (*Note:* If you have been assigned to care for multiple patients, you can click on **Return to Patient List** to select and review the report for each additional patient before going to the Nurses' Station.)

Note: Even though the Patient List is initially skipped when you sign in to work for Period of Care 4, you can still access this screen if you wish to review the shift-change report for any of the patients. To do so, simply click on **Patient List** near the top left corner of the Nurses' Station (or click on the clipboard to the left of the Kardex). Then click on **Get Report** for the patient(s) whose care you are reviewing. This may be done during any period of care.

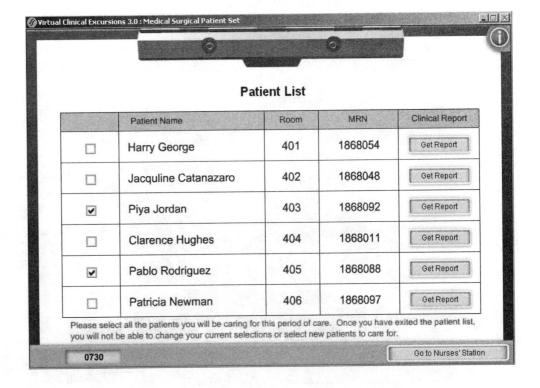

■ HOW TO FIND A PATIENT'S RECORDS

NURSES' STATION

Within the Nurses' Station, you will see:

1. A clipboard that contains the patient list for that floor.
2. A chart rack with patient charts labeled by room number, a notebook labeled Kardex, and a notebook labeled MAR (Medication Administration Record).
3. A desktop computer with access to the Electronic Patient Record (EPR).
4. A tool bar across the top of the screen that can also be used to access the Patient List, EPR, Chart, MAR, and Kardex. This tool bar is also accessible from each patient's room.
5. A Drug Guide containing information about the medications you are able to administer to your patients.
6. A tool bar across the bottom of the screen that you can use to access patient rooms, the Medication Room, the Floor Map, or the Drug Guide.

As you run your cursor over an item, it will be highlighted. To select, simply double-click on the item. As you use these resources, you will always be able to return to the Nurses' Station by clicking on the **Return to Nurses' Station** bar located in the right lower corner of your screen.

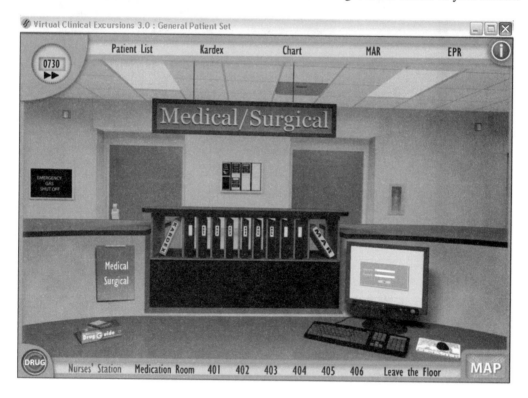

MEDICATION ADMINISTRATION RECORD (MAR)

The MAR icon located in the tool bar at the top of your screen accesses current 24-hour medications for each patient. Click on the icon and the MAR will open. (*Note:* You can also access the MAR by clicking on the MAR notebook on the far right side of the book rack in the center of the screen.) Within the MAR, tabs on the right side of the screen allow you to select patients by room number. Be careful to make sure you select the correct tab number for *your* patient rather than simply reading the first record that appears after the MAR opens. Each MAR sheet lists the following:

- Medications
- Route and dosage of each medication
- Times of administration of each medication

Note: The MAR changes each day. Expired MARs are stored in the patients' charts.

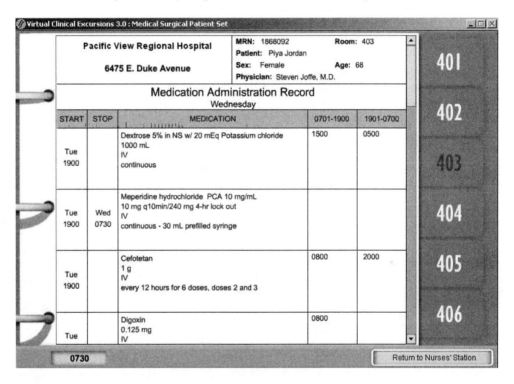

CHARTS

To access patient charts, either click on the **Chart** icon at the top of your screen or anywhere within the chart rack in the center of the Nurses' Station screen. When the close-up view appears, the individual charts are labeled by room number. To open a chart, click on the room number of the patient whose chart you wish to review. The patient's name and allergies will appear on the left side of the screen, along with a list of tabs on the right side of the screen, allowing you to view the following data:

- Allergies
- Physician's Orders
- Physician's Notes
- Nurse's Notes
- Laboratory Reports
- Diagnostic Reports
- Surgical Reports
- Consultations

- Patient Education
- History and Physical
- Nursing Admission
- Expired MARs
- Consents
- Mental Health
- Admissions
- Emergency Department

Information appears in real time. The entries are in reverse chronologic order, so use the down arrow at the right side of each chart page to scroll down to view previous entries. Flip from tab to tab to view multiple data fields or click on the **Return to Nurses' Station** bar in the lower right corner of the screen to exit the chart.

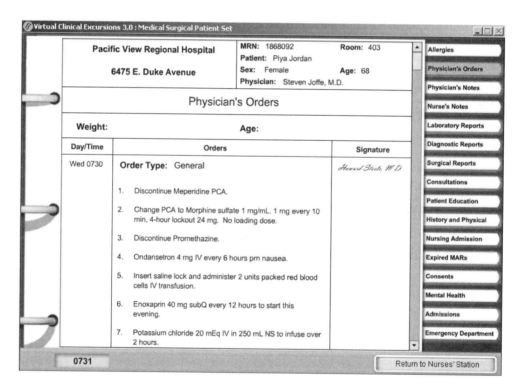

ELECTRONIC PATIENT RECORD (EPR)

The EPR can be accessed from the computer in the Nurses' Station or from the EPR icon located in the tool bar at the top of your screen. To access a patient's EPR:

- Click on either the computer screen or the **EPR** icon.
- Your username and password are automatically filled in.
- Click on **Login** to enter the EPR.
- *Note:* Like the MAR, the EPR is arranged numerically. Thus when you enter, you are initially shown the records of the patient in the lowest room number on the floor. To view the correct data for *your* patient, remember to select the correct room number, using the drop-down menu for the Patient field at the top left corner of the screen.

The EPR used in Pacific View Regional Hospital represents a composite of commercial versions being used in hospitals. You can access the EPR:

- to review existing data for a patient (by room number).
- to enter data you collect while working with a patient.

The EPR is updated daily, so no matter what day or part of a shift you are working, there will be a current EPR with the patient's data from the past days of the current hospital stay. This type of simulated EPR allows you to examine how data for different attributes have changed over time, as well as to examine data for all of a patient's attributes at a particular time. The EPR is fully functional (as it is in a real-life hospital). You can enter such data as blood pressure, breath sounds, and certain treatments. The EPR will not, however, allow you to enter data for a previous time period. Use the arrows at the bottom of the screen to move forward and backward in time.

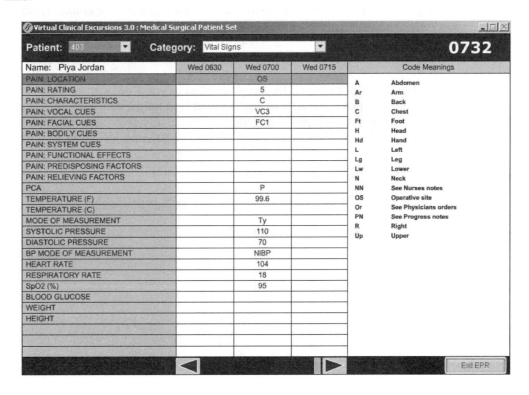

At the top of the EPR screen, you can choose patients by their room numbers. In addition, you have access to 17 different categories of patient data. To change patients or data categories, click the down arrow to the right of the room number or category.

The categories of patient data in the EPR as as follows:

- Vital Signs
- Respiratory
- Cardiovascular
- Neurologic
- Gastrointestinal
- Excretory
- Musculoskeletal
- Integumentary
- Reproductive
- Psychosocial
- Wounds and Drains
- Activity
- Hygiene and Comfort
- Safety
- Nutrition
- IV
- Intake and Output

Remember, each hospital selects its own codes. The codes used in the EPR at Pacific View Regional Hospital may be different from ones you have seen in your clinical rotations. Take some time to acquaint yourself with the codes. Within the Vital Signs category, click on any item in the left column (e.g., Pain: Characteristics). In the far-right column, you will see a list of code meanings for the possible findings and/or descriptors for that assessment area.

You will use the codes to record the data you collect as you work with patients. Click on the box in the last time column to the right of any item and wait for the code meanings applicable to that entry to appear. Select the appropriate code to describe your assessment findings and type it in the box. (*Note:* If no cursor appears within the box, click on the box again until the blue shading disappears and the blinking cursor appears.) Once the data are typed in this box, they are entered into the patient's record for this period of care only.

To leave the EPR, click on **Exit EPR** in the bottom right corner of the screen.

■ VISITING A PATIENT

From the Nurses' Station, click on the room number of the patient you wish to visit in the tool bar at the bottom of your screen. Once you are inside the room, you will see a still photo of your patient in the top left corner. To verify that this is the patient you have chosen, click on the **Check Armband** icon to the right of the photo. The patient's identification data will appear. If you click on **Check Allergies** (the next icon to the right), a list of the patient's allergies (if any) will replace the photo.

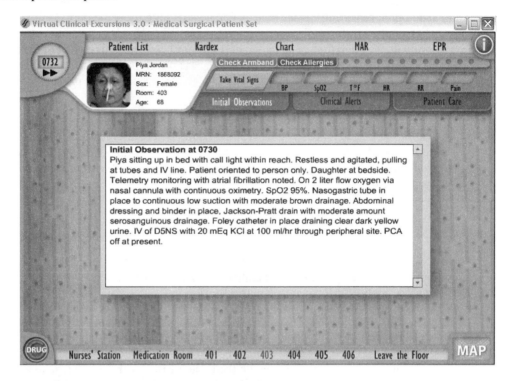

Also located in the patient's room are multiple icons you can use to assess the patient or the patient's medications. A virtual clock is provided in the upper left corner of the room to monitor your progress in real time. (*Note:* The fast forward icon within the virtual clock will advance the time by two-minute intervals when clicked.)

- The tool bar across the top of the screen allows you to check the **Patient List**, access the **EPR** to check or enter data, and view the patient's **Chart**, **MAR**, or **Kardex**.

- The **Take Vital Signs** icon allows you to measure the patient's up-to-the-minute blood pressure, oxygen saturation, temperature, heart rate, respiratory rate, and pain level.

- Each time you enter a patient's room, you are given an Initial Observation report to review (in the text box under the patient's photo). These notes are provided to give you a "look" at the patient as if you had just stepped into the room. You can also click on the **Initial Observations** icon to return to this box from other views within the patient's room. To the right of this icon is **Clinical Alerts**, a resource that allows you to make decisions about priority medication interventions based on emerging data collected in real time. Check this screen throughout your period of care to avoid missing critical information related to recently ordered or STAT medications.

- Clicking on the **Patient Care** icon opens up three specific learning environments within the patient room: **Physical Assessment**, **Nurse-Client Interactions**, and **Medication Administration**.

- To perform a **Physical Assessment**, choose a body area (such as **Head & Neck**) by clicking on the appropriate icon in the column of yellow buttons. This activates a list of system sub-categories for that body area (e.g., see **Sensory**, **Neurologic**, etc. in the green boxes). After you click on the system that you wish to evaluate, a still photo and text box appear, describing the assessment findings. The still photo is a "snapshot" of how an assessment of this area might be done or what the finding might look like. For every body area, there is also an **Equipment** button located on the far right of the screen.

- To the right of the Physical Assessment icon is **Nurse-Client Interactions**. Clicking on this icon will reveal the times and titles of any videos available for viewing. (*Note:* If the video you wish to see is not listed, this means you have not yet reached the correct virtual time to view that video. Check the virtual clock; you may return to access the video once its designated time has occurred—as long as you do so within the same period of care. Or you can click on the fast forward icon within the virtual clock to advance the time by two-minute intervals. You will then need to click on **Patient Care** and **Nurse-Client Interactions** again to refresh the screen.) To view a listed video, click on the white arrow to the right of the video title. Use the control buttons below the video to start, stop, pause, rewind, or fast-forward the action or to mute the sound.

- **Medication Administration** is the pathway that allows you to review and administer medications to a patient after you have prepared them in the Medication Room. This process is addressed further in the *How to Prepare Medications* section (pages 19-20) and in *Medications* (pages 26-30). For additional hands-on practice, see *Reducing Medication Errors* (pages 37-41).

▓ HOW TO QUIT, CHANGE PATIENTS, CHANGE FLOORS, OR CHANGE PERIOD OF CARE

How to Quit: From most screens, you may click the **Leave the Floor** icon on the bottom tool bar to the right of the patient room numbers. (*Note:* From some screens, you will first need to click an **Exit** button or **Return to Nurses' Station** before clicking **Leave the Floor**.) When the Floor Menu appears, click **Exit** to leave the program.

How to Change Patients, Floors, or Period of Care: To change patients, simply click on the new patient's room number. (You cannot receive a scorecard for a new patient, however, unless you have already selected that patient on the Patient List screen.) To change to a new period of care, to change floors, or to restart the virtual clock, click on **Leave the Floor** and then on **Restart the Program**.

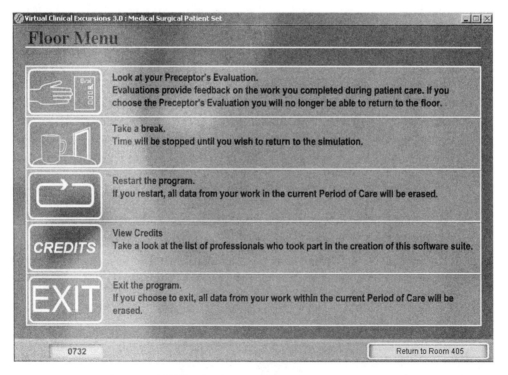

■ HOW TO PREPARE MEDICATIONS

From the Nurses' Station or the patient's room, you can access the Medication Room by clicking on the icon in the tool bar at the bottom of your screen to the left of the patient room numbers.

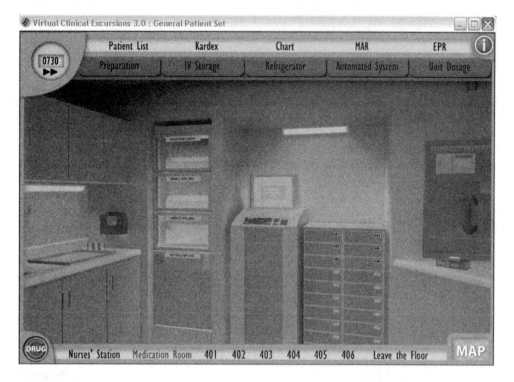

In the Medication Room you have access to the following (from left to right):

- A preparation area is located on the counter under the cabinets. To begin the medication preparation process, click on the tray on the counter or click on the **Preparation** icon at the top of the screen. The next screen leads you through a specific sequence (called the Preparation Wizard) to prepare medications one at a time for administration to a patient. However, no medication has been selected at this time. We will do this while working with a patient in *A Detailed Tour*. To exit this screen, click on **View Medication Room**.

- To the right of the cabinets (and above the refrigerator), IV storage bins are provided. Click on the bins themselves or on the **IV Storage** icon at the top of the screen. The bins are labeled **Microinfusion**, **Small Volume**, and **Large Volume**. Click on an individual bin to see a list of its contents. If you needed to prepare an IV medication at this time, you could click on the medication and its label would appear to the right under the patient's name. Next, you would click **Put Medication on Tray**. If you ever change your mind or choose the incorrect medication, you can reverse your actions by clicking on **Put Medication in Bin**. Click **Close Bin** in the right bottom corner to exit. **View Medication Room** brings you back to a full view of the entire room.

- A refrigerator is located under the IV storage bins to hold any medications that must be stored below room temperature. Click on the refrigerator door or on the **Refrigerator** icon at the top of the screen. Then click on the close-up view of the door to access the medications. When you are finished, click **Close Door** and then **View Medication Room**.

- To prepare controlled substances, click the **Automated System** icon at the top of the screen or click the computer monitor located to the right of the IV storage bins. A login screen will appear; your name and password are automatically filled in. Click **Login**. Select the patient for whom you wish to access medications; then select the correct medication drawer to open (they are stored alphabetically). Click **Open Drawer**, highlight the proper medication, and choose **Put Medication on Tray**. When you are finished, click **Close Drawer** and then **View Medication Room**.

- Next to the Automated System is a set of drawers identified by patient room number. To access these, click on the drawers themselves or on the **Unit Dosage** icon at the top of the screen. This provides a close-up view of the drawers. To open a drawer, click on the room number of the patient you are working with. Next, click on the medication you would like to prepare for the patient, and a label will appear to the right, listing the medication strength, units, and dosage per unit. You can **Open** and **Close** this medication label by clicking the appropriate icon. To exit, click **Close Drawer**; then click **View Medication Room**.

At any time, you can learn about a medication you wish to prepare for a patient by clicking on the **Drug** icon in the bottom left corner of the medication room screen or by clicking the **Drug Guide** book on the counter to the right of the unit dosage drawers. The **Drug Guide** provides information about the medications commonly included in nursing drug handbooks. Nutritional supplements and maintenance intravenous fluid preparations are not included.

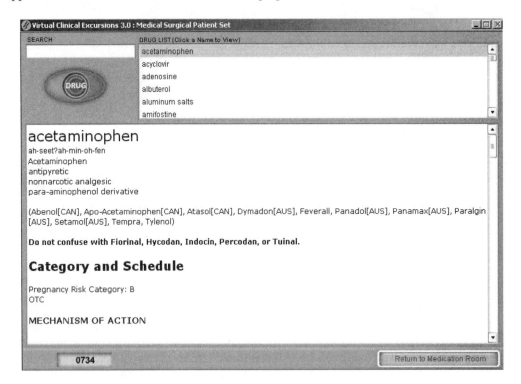

To access the MAR to review the medications ordered for a patient, click on the **MAR** icon located in the tool bar at the top of your screen and then click on the correct tab for your patient's room number. You may also click the **Review MAR** icon in the tool bar at the bottom of your screen from inside each medication storage area.

After you have chosen and prepared your medications, return to the patient's room to administer them by clicking on the room number in the bottom tool bar. Once inside the patient's room, click on **Patient Care** and then on **Medication Administration** and follow the proper administration sequence.

■ PRECEPTOR'S EVALUATIONS

When you have finished a session, click on **Leave the Floor** to go to the Floor Menu. At this point, you can click on the top icon (**Look at Your Preceptor's Evaluation**) to receive a score-card that provides feedback on the work you completed during patient care.

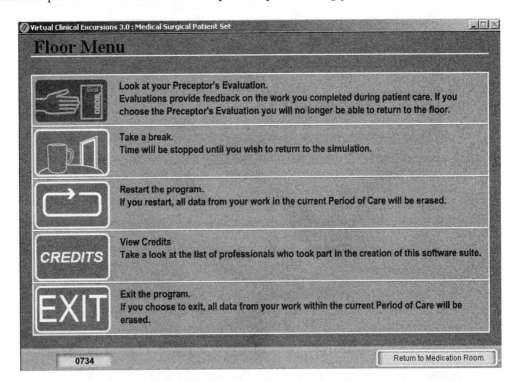

Evaluations are available for each patient you selected when you signed in for the current period of care. Click on the **Medication Scorecard** icon to see an example.

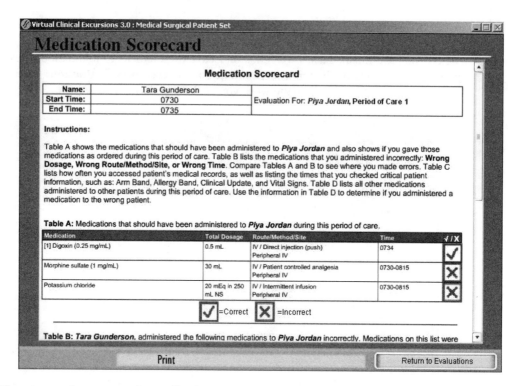

The scorecard compares the medications you administered to a patient during a period of care with what should have been administered. Table A lists the correct medications. Table B lists any medications that were administered incorrectly.

Remember, not every medication listed on the MAR should necessarily be given. For example, a patient might have an allergy to a drug that was ordered, or a medication might have been improperly transcribed to the MAR. Predetermined medication "errors" embedded within the program challenge you to exercise critical thinking skills and professional judgment when deciding to administer a medication, just as you would in a real hospital. Use all your available resources, such as the patient's chart and the MAR, to make your decision.

Table C lists the resources that were available to assist you in medication administration. It also documents whether and when you accessed these resources. For example, did you check the patient armband or perform a check of vital signs? If so, when?

You can click **Print** to get a copy of this report if needed. When you have finished reviewing the scorecard, click **Return to Evaluations** and then **Return to Menu**.

■ FLOOR MAP

To get a general sense of your location within the hospital, you can click on the **Map** icon found in the lower right corner of most of the screens in the *Virtual Clinical Excursions—General Hospital* program. (*Note:* If you are following this quick tour step by step, you will need to **Restart the Program** from the Floor Menu, sign in again, and go to the Nurses' Station to access the map.) When you click the **Map** icon, a floor map appears, showing the layout of the floor you are currently on, as well as a directory of the patients and services on that floor. As you move your cursor over the directory list, the location of each room is highlighted on the map (and vice versa). The floor map can be accessed from the Nurses' Station, Medication Room, and each patient's room.

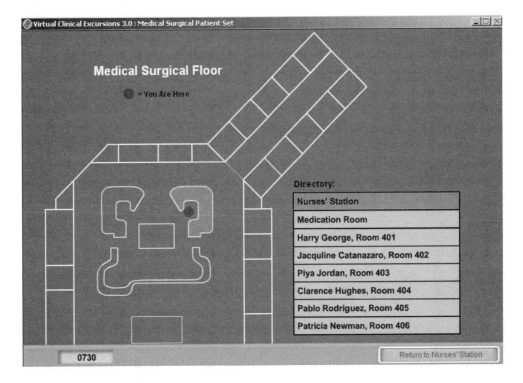

A DETAILED TOUR

If you wish to more thoroughly understand the capabilities of *Virtual Clinical Excursions—General Hospital*, take a detailed tour by completing the following section. During this tour, we will work with a specific patient to introduce you to all the different components and learning opportunities available within the software.

■ WORKING WITH A PATIENT

Sign in and select the Medical-Surgical floor for Period of Care 1 (0730-0815). From the Patient List, select Piya Jordan in Room 403; however, do not go to the Nurses' Station yet.

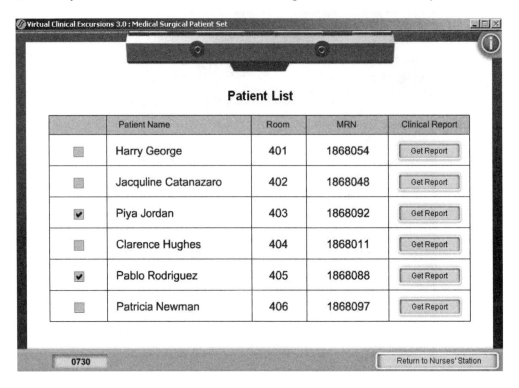

■ REPORT

In hospitals, when one shift ends and another begins, the outgoing nurse who attended a patient will give a verbal and sometimes a written summary of that patient's condition to the incoming nurse who will assume care for the patient. This summary is called a report and is an important source of data to provide an overview of a patient. Your first task is to get the clinical report on Piya Jordan. To do this, click **Get Report** in the far right column in this patient's row. From a brief review of this summary, identify the problems and areas of concern that you will need to address for this patient.

When you have finished noting any areas of concern, click on **Go to Nurses' Station**.

■ CHARTS

You can access Piya Jordan's chart from the Nurses' Station or from the patient's room (403). We will access it from the Nurses' Station: Click on the chart rack or on the **Chart** icon in the tool bar at the top of your screen. Next, click on the chart labeled **403** to open the medical record for Piya Jordan. Click on the **Emergency Department** tab to view a record of why this patient was admitted.

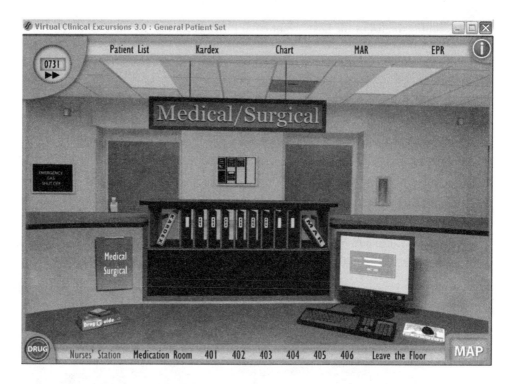

How many days has Piya Jordan been in the hospital?

What tests were done upon her arrival in the Emergency Department and why?

What was her reason for admission?

You should also click on **Surgical Reports** to learn what procedures were performed and when. Finally, review the **Nursing Admission** and **History and Physical** to learn about the health history of this patient. When you are done reviewing the chart, click **Return to Nurses' Station**.

■ MEDICATIONS

Open the Medication Administration Record (MAR) by clicking on the **MAR** icon in the tool bar at the top of your screen. *Remember:* The MAR automatically opens to the first occupied room number on the floor—which is not necessarily your patient's room number! Since you need to access Piya Jordan's MAR, click on tab **403** (her room number). Always make sure you are giving the *Right Drug to the Right Patient!*

Examine the list of medications ordered for Piya Jordan. In the table below, list the medications that need to be given during this period of care (0730-0815). For each medication, note the dosage, route, and time to be given.

Time	Medication	Dosage	Route

Click on **Return to Nurses' Station**. Next, click on **403** on the bottom tool bar and then verify that you are indeed in Piya Jordan's room. Select **Clinical Alerts** (the icon to the right of Initial Observations) to check for any emerging data that might affect your medication administration priorities. Next, go to the patient's chart (click on the **Chart** icon; then click on **403**). When the chart opens, select the **Physician's Orders** tab.

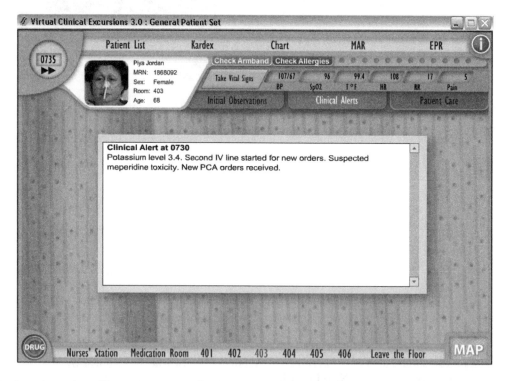

Review the orders. Have any new medications been ordered? Return to the MAR (click **Return to Room 403**; then click **MAR**). Verify that the new medications have been correctly transcribed to the MAR. Mistakes are sometimes made in the transcription process in the hospital setting, and it is sound practice to double-check any new order.

Are there any patient assessments you will need to perform before administering these medications? If so, return to Room 403 and click on **Patient Care** and then **Physical Assessment** to complete those assessments before proceeding.

Now click on the **Medication Room** icon in the tool bar at the bottom of your screen to locate and prepare the medications for Piya Jordan.

In the Medication Room, you must access the medications for Piya Jordan from the specific dispensing system in which each medication is stored. Locate each medication that needs to be given in this time period and click on **Put Medication on Tray** as appropriate. (*Hint:* Look in Unit Dosage drawer first.) When you are finished, click on **Close Drawer** and then on **View Medication Room**. Now click on the medication tray on the counter on the left side of the medication room screen to begin preparing the medications you have selected. (*Remember:* You can also click **Preparation** in the tool bar at the top of the screen.)

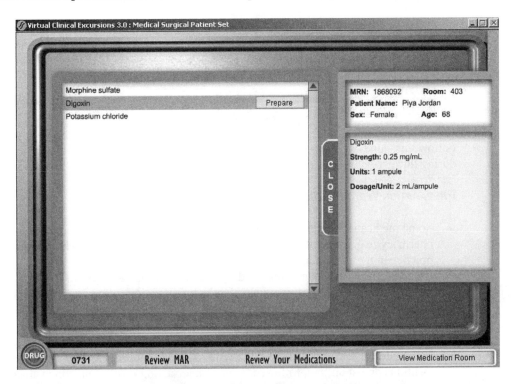

In the preparation area, you should see a list of the medications you put on the tray in the previous steps. Click on the first medication and then click **Prepare**. Follow the onscreen instructions of the Preparation Wizard, providing any data requested. As an example, let's follow the preparation process for digoxin, one of the medications due to be administered to Piya Jordan during this period of care. To begin, click to select **Digoxin**; then click **Prepare**. Now work through the Preparation Wizard sequence as detailed below:

Amount of medication in the ampule: 2 mL.
Enter the amount of medication you will draw up into a syringe: <u>**0.5**</u> mL.
Click **Next**.
Select the patient you wish to set aside the medication for: **Room 403, Piya Jordan**.
Click **Finish**.
Click **Return to Medication Room**.

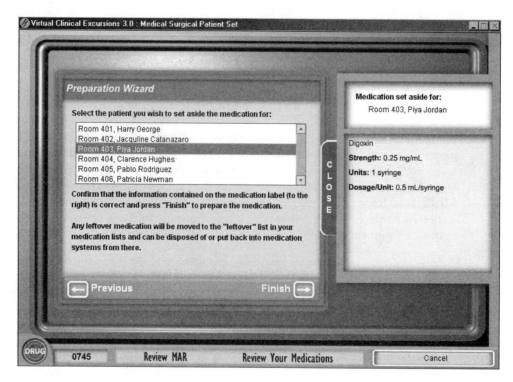

Follow this same basic process for the other medications due to be administered to Piya Jordan during this period of care. (*Hint:* Look in **IV Storage** and **Automated System**.)

PREPARATION WIZARD EXCEPTIONS

- Some medications in *Virtual Clinical Excursions—General Hospital* are prepared by the pharmacy (e.g., IV antibiotics) and taken to the patient room as a whole. This is common practice in most hospitals.
- Blood products are not administered by students through the *Virtual Clinical Excursions—General Hospital* simulations since blood administration follows specific protocols not covered in this program.
- The *Virtual Clinical Excursions—General Hospital* simulations do not allow for mixing more than one type of medication, such as regular and Lente insulins, in the same syringe. In the clinical setting, when multiple types of insulin are ordered for a patient, the regular insulin is drawn up first, followed by the longer-acting insulin. Insulin is always administered in a special unit-marked syringe.

Now return to Room 403 (click on **403** on the bottom tool bar) to administer Piya Jordan's medications.

At any time during the medication administration process, you can perform a further review of systems, take vital signs, check information contained within the chart, or verify patient identity and allergies. Inside Piya Jordan's room, click **Take Vital Signs**. (*Note:* These findings change over time to reflect the temporal changes you would find in a patient similar to Piya Jordan.)

When you have gathered all the data you need, click on **Patient Care** and then select **Medication Administration**. Any medications you prepared in the previous steps should be listed on the left side of your screen. Let's continue the administration process with the digoxin ordered for Piya Jordan. Click to highlight **Digoxin** in the list of medications. Next, click on the down arrow to the right of **Select** and choose **Administer** from the drop-down menu. This will activate the Administration Wizard. Complete the Wizard sequence as follows:

- Route: **IV**
- Method: **Direct Injection**
- Site: **Peripheral IV**
- Click **Administer to Patient** arrow.
- Would you like to document this administration in the MAR? **Yes**
- Click **Finish** arrow.

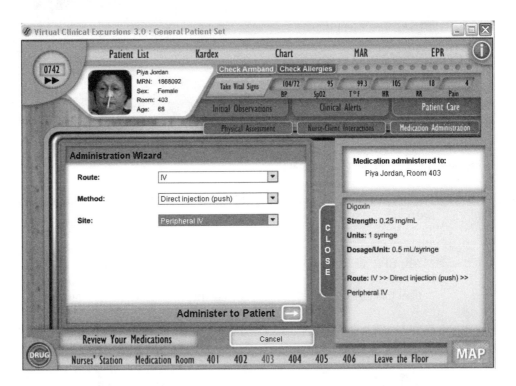

Your selections are recorded by a tracking system and evaluated on a Medication Scorecard stored under Preceptor's Evaluations. This scorecard can be viewed, printed, and given to your instructor. To access the Preceptor's Evaluations, click on **Leave the Floor**. When the Floor Menu appears, click on the icon next to **Look at Your Preceptor's Evaluation**. Then click on **Medication Scorecard** inside the box with Piya Jordan's name (see example on the following page).

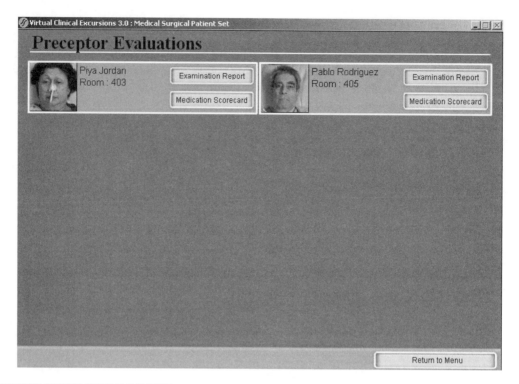

■ MEDICATION SCORECARD

- First, review Table A. Was digoxin given correctly? Did you give the other medications as ordered?
- Table B shows you which (if any) medications you gave incorrectly.
- Table C addresses the resources used for Piya Jordan. Did you access the patient's chart, MAR, EPR, or Kardex as needed to make safe medication administration decisions?
- Did you check the patient's armband to verify her identity? Did you check whether your patient had any known allergies to medications? Were vital signs taken?

When you have finished reviewing the scorecard, click **Return to Evaluations** and then **Return to Menu**.

■ VITAL SIGNS

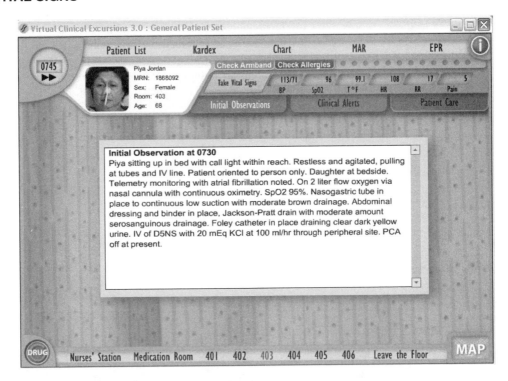

Vital signs, often considered the traditional "signs of life," include body temperature, heart rate, respiratory rate, blood pressure, oxygen saturation of the blood, and pain level.

Inside Piya Jordan's room, click **Take Vital Signs**. (*Note:* If you are following this detailed tour step by step, you will need to **Restart the Program** from the Floor Menu, sign in again, and navigate to Room 403.) Collect vital signs for this patient and record them in the following table. Note the time at which you collected each of these data. (*Remember:* You can take vital signs at any time. The data change over time to reflect the temporal changes you would find in a patient similar to Piya Jordan.)

Vital Signs	Findings/Time
Blood pressure	
O$_2$ saturation	
Heart rate	
Respiratory rate	
Temperature	
Pain rating	

After you are done, click on the **EPR** icon located in the tool bar at the top of the screen. Your username and password are automatically provided. Click on **Login** to enter the EPR. To access Piya Jordan's records, click on the down arrow next to Patient and choose her room number, **403**. Select **Vital Signs** as the category. Next, in the empty time column on the far right, record the vital signs data you just collected in Piya Jordan's room. (*Note:* If you need help with this process, see page 16.) Now compare these findings with the data you collected earlier for this patient's vital signs. Use these earlier findings to establish a baseline for each of the vital signs.

a. Are any of the data you collected significantly different from the baseline for a particular vital sign?

Circle One: Yes No

b. If "Yes," which data are different?

PHYSICAL ASSESSMENT

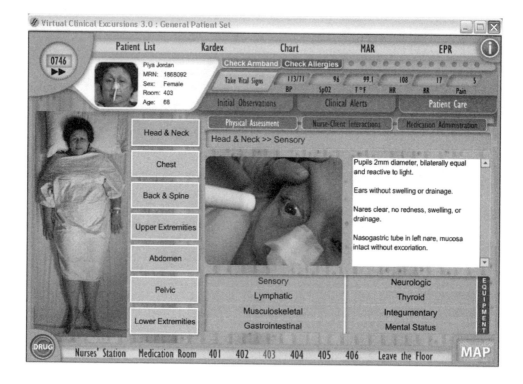

After you have finished examining the EPR for vital signs, click **Exit EPR** to return to Room 403. Click **Patient Care** and then **Physical Assessment**. Think about what information you received in the report at the beginning of this shift, as well as what you may have learned about this patient from the chart. Based on this, what area(s) of examination should you pay most attention to at this time? Is there any equipment you should be monitoring? Conduct a physical assessment of the body areas and systems that you consider priorities for Piya Jordan. For example, select **Head & Neck**; then click on and assess **Sensory** and **Lymphatic**. Complete any other assessment(s) you think are necessary at this time. In the following table, record the data you collected during this examination.

Area of Examination	Findings
Head & Neck Sensory	
Head & Neck Lymphatic	

After you have finished collecting these data, return to the EPR. Compare the data that were already in the record with those you just collected.

a.   Are any of the data you collected significantly different from the baselines for this patient?

Circle One: Yes   No

b.   If "Yes," which data are different?

■ **NURSE-CLIENT INTERACTIONS**

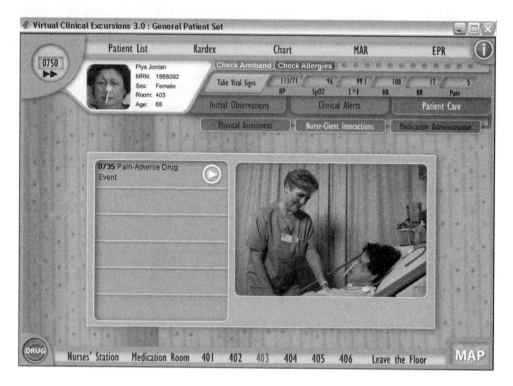

Click on **Patient Care** from inside Piya Jordan's room (403). Now click on **Nurse-Client Interactions** to access a short video titled **Pain—Adverse Drug Event**, which is available for viewing at or after 0735 (based on the virtual clock in the upper left corner of your screen; see *Note* below.). To begin the video, click on the arrow next to its title. You will observe a nurse communicating with Piya Jordan and her daughter. There are many variations of nursing practice, some exemplifying "best" practice and some not. Note whether the nurse in this interaction displays professional behavior and compassionate care. Are her words congruent with what is going on with the patient? Does this interaction "feel right" to you? If not, how would you handle this situation differently? Explain.

Note: If the video you wish to view is not listed, this means you have not yet reached the correct virtual time to view that video. Check the virtual clock; you may return to access the video once its designated time has occurred—as long as you do so within the same period of care. Or you can click on the fast forward icon within the virtual clock to advance the time by two-minute intervals. You will then need to click on **Patient Care** and **Nurse-Client Interactions** again to refresh the screen.

At least one Nurse-Client Interactions video is available during each period of care. Viewing these videos can help you learn more about what is occurring with a patient at a certain time and also prompt you to discern between nurse communications that are ideal and those that need improvement. Compassionate care and the ability to communicate clearly are essential components of delivering quality nursing care, and it is during your clinical time that you will begin to refine these skills.

■ COLLECTING AND EVALUATING DATA

Each of the activities you perform in the Patient Care environment generates a significant amount of assessment data. Remember that after you collect data, you can record your findings in the EPR. You can also review the EPR, patient's chart, videos, and MAR at any time. You will get plenty of practice collecting and then evaluating data in context of the patient's course.

Now, here's an important question for you:

> Did the previous sequence of exercises provide the most efficient way to assess Piya Jordan?

For example, you went to the patient's room to get vital signs, then back to the EPR to enter data and compare your findings with extant data. Next, you went back to the patient's room to do a physical examination, then again back to the EPR to enter and review data. If this back-and-forth process of data collection and recording seemed inefficient, remember the following:

- Plan all of your nursing activities to maximize efficiency, while at the same time optimizing the quality of patient care. (Think about what data you might need before performing certain tasks. For example, do you need to check a heart rate before administering a cardiac medication or check an IV site before starting an infusion?)

- You collect a tremendous amount of data when you work with a patient. Very few people can accurately remember all these data for more than a few minutes. Develop efficient assessment skills, and record data as soon as possible after collecting them.

- Assessment data are only the starting point for the nursing process.

Make a clear distinction between these first exercises and how you actually provide nursing care. These initial exercises were designed to involve you actively in the use of different software components. This workbook focuses on sensible practices for implementing the nursing process in ways that ensure the highest-quality care of patients.

Most important, remember that a human being changes through time, and that these changes include both the physical and psychosocial facets of a person as a living organism. Think about this for a moment. Some patients may change physically in a very short time (a patient with emerging myocardial infarction) or more slowly (a patient with a chronic illness). Patients' overall physical and psychosocial conditions may improve or deteriorate. They may have effective coping skills and familial support, or they may feel alone and full of despair. In fact, each individual is a complex mix of physical and psychosocial elements, and at least some of these elements usually change through time.

Thus it is crucial that you *DO NOT* think of the nursing process as a simple one-time, five-step procedure consisting of assessment, nursing diagnosis, planning, implementation, and evaluation. Rather, the nursing process should be utilized as a creative and systematic approach to delivering nursing care. Furthermore, because all living organisms are constantly changing, we must apply the nursing process over and over. Each time we follow the nursing process for an individual patient, we refine our understanding of that patient's physical and psychosocial conditions based on collection and analysis of many different types of data. *Virtual Clinical Excursions—General Hospital* will help you develop both the creativity and the systematic approach needed to become a nurse who is equipped to deliver the highest-quality care to all patients.

REDUCING MEDICATION ERRORS

Earlier in this detailed tour, you learned the basic steps of medication preparation and administration. The following simulations will allow you to practice those skills further—with an increased emphasis on reducing medication errors by using the Medication Scorecard to evaluate your work.

Sign in to work at Pacific View Regional Hospital for Period of Care 1. (*Note:* If you are already working with another patient or during another period of care, click on **Leave the Floor** and then **Restart the Program**; then sign in.)

From the Patient List, select Clarence Hughes. Then click on **Go to Nurses' Station**. Complete the following steps to prepare and administer medications to Clarence Hughes.

- Click on **Medication Room**.
- Click on **MAR** and then on tab **404** to determine prn medications that have been ordered for Clarence Hughes to address his constipation and pain. (*Note:* You may click on **Review MAR** at any time to verify the correct medication order. Always remember to check the patient name on the MAR to make sure you have the correct patient's record—you must click on the correct room number tab within the MAR.) Click on **Return to Medication Room** after reviewing the correct MAR.
- Click on **Unit Dosage** (or on the Unit Dosage cabinet); from the close-up view, click on drawer **404**.
- Select the medications you would like to administer. After each selection, click **Put Medication on Tray**. When you are finished selecting medications, click **Close Drawer** and then **View Medication Room**.
- Click **Automated System** (or on the Automated System unit itself). Click **Login**.
- On the next screen, specify the correct patient and drawer location.
- Select the medication you would like to administer and click **Put Medication on Tray**. Repeat this process if you wish to administer other medications from the Automated System.
- When you are finished, click **Close Drawer** and **View Medication Room**.
- From the Medication Room, click **Preparation** (or on the preparation tray).
- From the list of medications on your tray, highlight the correct medication to administer and click **Prepare**.
- This activates the Preparation Wizard. Supply any requested information; then click **Next**.
- Now select the correct patient to receive this medication and click **Finish**.
- Repeat the previous three steps until all medications that you want to administer are prepared.
- You can click on **Review Your Medications** and then on **Return to Medication Room** when ready. Once you are back in the Medication Room, go directly to Clarence Hughes' room by clicking on **404** at the bottom of the screen.
- Inside the patient's room, administer the medication, utilizing the five rights of medication administration. After you have collected the appropriate assessment data and are ready for administration, click **Patient Care** and then **Medication Administration**. Verify that the correct patient and medication(s) appear in the left-hand window. Highlight the first medication you wish to administer; then click the down arrow next to Select. From the drop-down menu, select **Administer** and complete the Administration Wizard by providing any information requested. When the Wizard stops asking for information, click **Administer to Patient**. Specify **Yes** when asked whether this administration should be recorded in the MAR. Finally, click **Finish**.

■ **SELF-EVALUATION**

Now let's see how you did during your medication administration!

- Click on **Leave the Floor** at the bottom of your screen. From the Floor Menu, select **Look at Your Preceptor's Evaluation**. Then click **Medication Scorecard**.

These resources will help you find out more about each patient's medications and possible sources of medication errors.

1. Start by examining Table A. These are the medications you should have given to Clarence Hughes during this period of care. If each of the medications in Table A has a ✓ by it, then you made no errors. Congratulations!

If any medication has an X by it, then you made one or more medication errors.

Compare Tables A and B to determine which of the following types of errors you made: Wrong Dose, Wrong Route/Method/Site, or Wrong Time. Follow these steps:
   a. Find medications in Table A that were given incorrectly.
   b. Now see if those same medications are in Table B, which shows what you actually administered to Clarence Hughes.
   c. Comparing Tables A and B, match the Strength, Dose, Route/Method/Site, and Time for each medication you administered incorrectly.
   d. Then, using the form below, list the medications given incorrectly and mark the errors you made for each medication.

Medication	Strength	Dosage	Route	Method	Site	Time
	❏	❏	❏	❏	❏	❏
	❏	❏	❏	❏	❏	❏
	❏	❏	❏	❏	❏	❏
	❏	❏	❏	❏	❏	❏

2. To help you reduce future medication errors, consider the following list of possible reasons for errors.

- Did not check drug against MAR for correct patient, correct date, correct time, correct drug, and correct dose.
- Did not check drug dose against MAR three times.
- Did not open the unit dose package in the patient's room.
- Did not correctly identify the patient using two identifiers.
- Did not administer the drug on time.
- Did not verify patient allergies.
- Did not check the patient's current condition or vital sign parameters.
- Did not consider why the patient would be receiving this drug.
- Did not question why the drug was in the patient's drawer.
- Did not check the physician's order and/or check with the pharmacist when there was a question about the drug or dose.
- Did not verify that no adverse effects had occurred from a previous dose.

Based on these possibilities, determine how you made each error and record the reason into the form below:

Medication	Reason for Error

3. Look again at Table B. Are there medications listed that are not in Table A? If so, you gave a medication to Clarence Hughes that he should not have received. Complete the following exercises to help you understand how such an error might have been made.

   a. Perhaps you gave a medication that was on Clarence Hughes' MAR for this period of care, without recognizing that a change had occurred in the patient's condition, which should have caused you to reconsider. Review patient records as necessary and complete the following form:

Medication	Possible Reasons Not to Give This Medication

   b. Another possibility is that you gave Clarence Hughes a medication that should have been given at a different time. Check his MAR and complete the form below to determine whether you made a Wrong Time error:

Medication	Given to Clarence Hughes at What Time	Should Have Been Given at What Time

c. Maybe you gave another patient's medication to Clarence Hughes. In this case, you made a Wrong Patient error. Check the MARs of other patients and use the form below to determine whether you made this type of error:

Medication	Given to Clarence Hughes	Should Have Been Given to

4. The Medication Scorecard provides some other interesting sources of information. For example, if there is a medication selected for Clarence Hughes but it was not given to him, there will be an X by that medication in Table A, but it will not appear in Table B. In that case, you might have given this medication to some other patient, which is another type of Wrong Patient error. To investigate further, look at Table D, which lists the medications you gave to other patients. See whether you can find any medications for Clarence Hughes that were given to another patient by mistake. However, before you make any decisions, be sure to cross-check the MAR for other patients because the same medication may have been ordered for multiple patients. Use the following form to record your findings:

Medication	Should Have Been Given to Clarence Hughes	Given by Mistake to

5. Now take some time to review the medication exercises you just completed. Use the form below to create an overall analysis of what you have learned. Once again, record each of the medication errors you made, including the type of each error. Then, for each error you made, indicate specifically what you would do differently to prevent this type of error from occurring again.

Medication	Type of Error	Error Prevention Tactic

Submit this form to your instructor if required as a graded assignment, or simply use these exercises to improve your understanding of medication errors and how to reduce them.

Name: _____   Date: _____

The following icons are used throughout the workbook to help you quickly identify particular activities and assignments:

 Indicates a reading assignment—tells you which textbook chapter(s) you should read before starting each lesson

 Indicates a writing activity

 Marks the beginning of an interactive CD-ROM activity—signals you to open or return to your *Virtual Clinical Excursions—General Hospital* CD-ROM

 Indicates additional CD-ROM instructions

 Indicates questions and activities that require you to consult your textbook

 Indicates the approximate time required to complete an exercise

LESSON 1

Critical Thinking and Problem Solving

/◌◌◌ **Reading Assignment:** Overview of the Nursing Process and Critical Thinking (Chapter 4)

Assessment, Nursing Diagnosis, and Planning (Chapter 5)

Assisting with Respiration and Oxygen Delivery (Chapter 28)

Patient: Patricia Newman, Medical-Surgical Floor, Room 406

Objectives:

- Use critical thinking to gather and analyze data presented in the case study.
- Use the problem-solving process to decide which assessment data are needed to provide appropriate nursing care for a patient.
- Use critical thinking in order to organize tasks and set priorities.

The directed, purposeful activity by which assessment is performed, data are gathered and analyzed, and care plans are constructed is a good example of critical thinking. Decisions are made regarding what components of physical assessment ("focused assessment") are most essential for a particular patient at a given time. Orderly, systematic chart review provides data that combine with physical assessment findings to support nursing diagnoses. Decisions can then be made to choose the best actions to meet a particular goal.

Exercise 1

 CD-ROM Activity—Gathering Data

 15 minutes

- Sign in to work at Pacific View Regional Hospital on the Medical-Surgical Floor for Period of Care 1. (*Note:* If you are already in the virtual hospital from a previous exercise, click on **Leave the Floor** and then **Restart the Program** to get to the sign-in window.)
- From the Patient List, select Patricia Newman (Room 406).
- Click on **Get Report** for Patricia Newman and take notes as needed.

1. Fill in the following form as you obtain report on Patricia Newman:

Respiratory status:

Vital signs: BP _____ HR _____ RR _____ T _____ SpO$_2$ _____

IV:

Priority problem:

Diagnostic tests:

→ • Click on **Go to Nurses' Station**.

2. From the list below, select and mark with an X those sections of Patricia Newman's patient records you will need to consult at this time to gather necessary data to safely care for her. (*Hint:* See page 57 in your textbook.)

_____ a. Admissions Records

_____ b. Operative Reports

_____ c. Nursing History

_____ d. Medication Records

_____ e. History & Physical

_____ f. Social Services

_____ g. Physician's Notes

_____ h. Nurse's Notes

_____ i. Diagnostic Reports

_____ j. Kardex

_____ k. Physician's Orders

• Click on **Kardex** at the top of the screen. Click on tab **406** and read Patricia Newman's records. (*Remember:* The Kardex provides access to the records of all patients on the floor—not just the patient for whom you are currently caring. Be sure you are looking at the Kardex for the correct room number!)

3. Does Patricia Newman have any allergies that are pertinent to your care for her? (*Hint:* Allergies are listed after the patient problems in the Kardex.)

4. What categories of problems are marked "initiated" on Patricia Newman's Kardex?

5. What are Patricia Newman's diagnoses as listed on the Kardex?

6. Indicate which area is the priority problem for Patricia Newman at this time. Mark your choice with an X.

_____ a. Movement and activity

_____ b. Circulation

_____ c. Airway and breathing

_____ d. Safety

_____ e. Security

_____ f. Elimination

Exercise 2

CD-ROM Activity—Priority Assessments and Pulse Oximetry

30 minutes

Read in your textbook about pneumonia and emphysema (COPD).

- Sign in to work at Pacific View Regional Hospital on the Medical-Surgical Floor for Period of Care 1. (*Note:* If you are already in the virtual hospital from a previous exercise, click on **Leave the Floor** and then **Restart the Program** to get to the sign-in window.)
- From the Patient List, select Patricia Newman (Room 406).
- Click on **Go to Nurses' Station**.
- Click on **Chart** and then on the chart for Room **406**.
- Click on **Laboratory Tests**. Read the blood count report.

1. Patricia Newman's white blood cell count is _____. This is _____ (consistent/inconsistent) with her diagnosis of pneumonia.

2. Considering Patricia Newman's respiratory status and problems, determine assessments that should be performed during your first visit to the patient. From the list below, mark with an X those areas you would assess on the first visit to Patricia Newman.

    _____ a. Vital signs

    _____ b. Verbal complaints

    _____ c. Heart

    _____ d. Lungs

    _____ e. IV

    _____ f. Eyes

    _____ g. Pain level

    _____ h. Skin

    _____ i. Extremities

    _____ j. Abdomen

    _____ k. Neurologic status

• Click on **Return to Nurses' Station**.
• Now click on **406** at the bottom of your screen to go to Patricia Newman's room.
• Click on **Initial Observations**, read the note, and then click on **Clinical Alerts**.

3. What two problems are identified in the initial observation and the clinical alert? (*Hint:* What is the normal range for SpO_2? See page 495 in your textbook.)

4. Normal oxygen saturation is _____.

• Click on **Check Armband** and then on **Take Vital Signs**.

5. Record Patricia Newman's vital sign measurements below. (*Note:* You will need to enter them in the EPR later.)

BP _____ T _____ SpO_2 _____ HR _____ RR _____ Pain level _____

Read about pulse oximetry on pages 495-497 in your textbook.

6. How does the pulse oximeter measure oxygen saturation?

7. Is there a problem with using a fingertip probe for pulse oximetry if the patient is wearing nail polish or artificial nails?

8. If you didn't want to use Patricia Newman's finger for the pulse oximeter probe, where would you place it?

→ • Click on **Patient Care** and then on **Chest**.
   • Click on **Respiratory** and note the respiratory assessment data.
   • Click on the **Musculoskeletal** subcategory of the respiratory assessment and note the data that are pertinent regarding respiration.

9. Record the respiratory assessment findings below.

Read about pneumonia in your medical-surgical textbook.

→ • Click on **Chart** and then on **406**.
   • Click on **Laboratory Tests**. Read the blood count report (CBC).
   • Click on **Diagnostic Reports** and read the x-ray report from Tuesday.

10. Which signs and symptoms of pneumonia does Patricia Newman have? Mark your choice(s) with an X.

_____ a. Elevated blood pressure

_____ b. Impaired respiration

_____ c. Tachycardia

_____ d. Crackles in lungs

_____ e. Elevated white blood cell count

_____ f. Infiltrates on x-ray

_____ g. Fever

_____ h. Tachypnea

_____ i. Diminished aeration

→ • Click on **Return to Room 406**.
   • Click on **EPR** and then on **Login**.
   • In the Patient box in the upper left-hand corner of the screen, choose **406** from the drop-down menu. Verify that the page is for Patricia Newman. Keep **Vital Signs** as the category.
   • In the correct column enter the pain rating and vital signs you recorded in question 5 of this exercise.
   • Now click on the arrow to the right of the Category box at the top of the screen. Choose **Respiratory**. Enter the data you obtained when that system was assessed in question 9.
   • Click on the various lines where data are entered to highlight and view the codes used for charting about that part of the system. (*Hint:* The code meanings are listed to the right of the data columns.)

11. What differences did you find between what you have charted and what was charted for these systems on Wednesday at 0300?

Exercise 3

CD-ROM Activity—Problem Solving and Prioritizing

30 minutes

• Sign in to work at Pacific View Regional Hospital on the Medical-Surgical Floor for Period of Care 1. (*Note:* If you are already in the virtual hospital from a previous exercise, click on **Leave the Floor** and then **Restart the Program** to get to the sign-in window.)
• From the Patient List, select **Patricia Newman** (Room 406).
• Click on **Go to Nurses' Station**.

1. Indicate which area is the priority problem for Patricia Newman at this time. Mark your choice with an X.

_____ a. Movement and activity

_____ b. Circulation

_____ c. Airway and oxygenation

_____ d. Safety

_____ e. Security

→ • Click on **Chart** and then on the chart for **406**.

• Click on the chart tab for **History and Physical** and read the records.

2. How many times has Patricia Newman been hospitalized for pneumonia in the past 2 years?

3. What do you think are contributing factors for this problem?

4. You will be expected to do discharge teaching for Patricia Newman during her hospital stay. How would you approach the topic of recurrent pneumonia? Select the actions below that you think would work best for her and number them in the order in which you would use them.

_____   a. Give the patient smoking cessation literature to read.

_____   b. Find out how she feels about the repeated hospitalizations.

_____   c. Ask whether she has ever tried to quit smoking.

_____   d. Explain how smoking predisposes her to lung infection.

_____   e. Provide a list of community resources for quitting smoking.

 5. What actions can you teach Patricia Newman to do at home that will help to keep her lungs clear? (*Hint:* Review pneumonia and nursing interventions in your medical-surgical text-book.)

LESSON 2

Priority Setting

 Reading Assignment: Concepts of Health, Illness, and Health Promotion (Chapter 2)
Overview of the Nursing Process and Critical Thinking
(Chapter 4)
Assessment, Nursing Diagnosis, and Planning (Chapter 5)
Concepts of Basic Nutrition and Cultural Considerations
(Chapter 26)

Patient: Patricia Newman, Medical-Surgical Floor, Room 406

Objectives:

- Prioritize nursing diagnoses in order of importance for a patient's well-being.
- Prioritize tasks appropriately.

Priority setting is a skill that each nurse must develop in order to work efficiently and safely.
Along with prioritization is the need to recognize when delegation is necessary. Appropriate delegation is essential for the safety of patients. One must be certain that the person to whom a task is delegated is capable of performing the task safely and effectively. Learning what tasks can be delegated to the CNAs is essential wherever one works.

Exercise 1

 CD-ROM Activity—Problems and Nursing Diagnoses

30 minutes

- Sign in to work at Pacific View Regional Hospital on the Medical-Surgical Floor for Period of Care 3. (*Note:* If you are already in the virtual hospital from a previous exercise, click on **Leave the Floor** and then **Restart the Program** to get to the sign-in window.)
- From the Patient List, select Patricia Newman (Room 406).
- Click on **Get Report** for Patricia Newman and take notes as needed.
- Click on **Go to Nurses' Station**.
- Click on **EPR** and then on the **Login** button.
- In the Patient box, choose **406** from the drop-down menu.
- In the Category box, select **Intake and Output**.
- Use the arrows at the bottom of the screen to scroll back and forth in time.

1. Calculate the total intake and output for Wednesday. Patricia Newman's total intake for

   Wednesday is _____. Her total output is _____.

→ • Change the Category to **Nutrition** and scroll back and forth to review data.

2. Patricia Newman ate _____% of her breakfast and _____% of her lunch.

→ • Click on **Exit EPR**.
  • Next, click on **Chart** and then on **406**.
  • Click on **Consultations** and read the dietary consult.

3. What are the dietary recommendations made by the dietitian?

4. Below, match each NANDA nursing diagnosis with the related problem area.

Problem	**Nursing Diagnosis**
_____ Discharge	a. Gas exchange, impaired
_____ Fluid/volume electrolyte imbalance	b. Deficient knowledge
_____ Infection	c. Nutrition, less than body requirements
_____ Nutrition	d. Hyperthermia
_____ Respiratory	e. Infection (risk for)
_____ Thermoregulation	f. Fluid volume, risk for imbalanced

There is not always a clear-cut or appropriate NANDA nursing diagnosis for every problem. The list is still evolving. For this reason, some hospitals use a problem list rather than a nursing diagnosis list.

5. Match the following data with the nursing diagnosis they support.

Nursing Diagnosis	**Data**
_____ Gas exchange, impaired	a. Eating 30%-40% of meals
_____ Nutrition, less than body requirements	b. Potassium 3.2 mEq/L
_____ Infection (risk for)	c. Temperature 102.5° F
_____ Fluid volume, risk for imbalance	d. Crackles in lower lobes of lungs
_____ Deficient knowledge	e. Is removing nasal oxygen cannula
_____ Hyperthermia	f. White blood cell count 16,000 mm^3
	g. Smokes cigarettes

Often a piece of data may fit with more than one nursing diagnosis. Nurses often consolidate the nursing diagnoses. For example, "coughing yellow sputum," "WBCs 16,000 mm^3," and "temperature 102.5° F" could be placed with the nursing diagnosis of Impaired gas exchange rather than Infection (risk for). Patricia Newman's pneumonia is what is contributing to her impaired gas exchange, along with her long-standing and worsening emphysema. It is a requirement that every nursing diagnosis or problem in the care plan be addressed in documentation at least once in 24 hours. When there are slim data, it is often expedient to place the data with a higher-priority nursing diagnosis/problem.

6. Choose the three nursing diagnoses that you feel represent Patricia Newman's most important problems.

7. Now, considering the data that support the nursing diagnoses you identified above, place the nursing diagnoses in order of priority. (*Hint:* Consider Maslow's Hierarchy of Needs, page 16 in the textbook, as well as what seems most important to the patient.)

Exercise 2

 CD-ROM Activity—Priorities Based on Maslow's Hierarchy

 30 minutes

- Sign in to work at Pacific View Regional Hospital on the Medical-Surgical Floor for Period of Care 3. (*Note:* If you are already in the virtual hospital from a previous exercise, click on **Leave the Floor** and then **Restart the Program** to get to the sign-in window.)
- From the Patient List, select Patricia Newman (Room 406).
- Click on **Go to Nurses' Station** and then **406** at the bottom of the screen.
- Read the Initial Observation.
- Click **Chart** and then on **406**; select the tab for **Nursing Admission**.
- Read through this record and note pertinent data in the spaces below. (*Hint:* Look for data that support the nursing diagnoses.)

  1. a. What is her height? _____

     b. What is her weight? _____

     c. What is her age? _____

  2. Do you think that Patricia Newman's weight is appropriate for her height and age?

 • Click on the **Laboratory Reports** tab of the chart.
  - Note the laboratory values for the various tests.

  3. Which tests result would be the most important to know considering Patricia Newman's diagnosis of pneumonia?

4. Besides the fact that Patricia Newman is eating only small portions of her meals, what other data that you've gathered support the nursing diagnosis of Nutrition, less than body requirements? Mark an X next to any data that would support this diagnosis. (*Hint:* Compare the laboratory values in the chart with normal ranges as listed in Appendix 4 of your textbook. Also, check Table 26-10 on page 459. Finally, review the data you gathered in Lesson 1.)

_____ a. 5 ft 5 in tall; weight 120 lb

_____ b. RBCs 4.9

_____ c. Hematocrit 45

_____ d. Fatigues easily

_____ e. Has frequent infections

_____ f. Needs supplemental oxygen

5. Considering the dietitian's recommendations, Patricia Newman's respiratory status, and her diagnosis of pneumonia, mark with an X the action that would be the first priority for her. (*Hint:* Read about pneumonia in your medical-surgical textbook if you need help.)

_____ a. Explain the importance of keeping the oxygen cannula in place.

_____ b. Return the oxygen cannula to her nose.

_____ c. Encourage her to drink 8 oz of water.

_____ d. Assess what liquids she finds appealing.

_____ e. Discuss why she should eat more of her meals.

6. Now mark an X by the action that would be the next priority action for Patricia Newman.

_____ a. Explain the importance of keeping the oxygen cannula in place.

_____ b. Return the oxygen cannula to her nose.

_____ c. Encourage her to drink 8 oz of water.

_____ d. Assess what liquids she finds appealing.

_____ e. Discuss why she should eat more of her meals.

 7. Oxygen and nutrition are considered to be _____ needs by Maslow. (*Hint:* see page 16 in your textbook.)

8. Which of the following would be considered first-level needs according to Maslow? Mark the correct choice(s) with an X.

_____ a. Hygiene

_____ b. Rest and comfort

_____ c. Psychologic comfort

_____ d. Affection

_____ e. Activity

_____ f. Elimination

_____ g. Safety

_____ h. Sexual procreation

_____ i. Intimacy

_____ j. Achievement

_____ k. Learning

Remember: When prioritizing nursing diagnoses, you must consider what is most important to the patient as well as what problem might be a threat to the patient's safety or well-being. Almost invariably, airway takes precedence over any other need. Safety, especially in a health care facility, is a high priority. Pain is another high priority.

Applying the Nursing Process

Reading Assignment: Overview of the Nursing Process and Critical Thinking
(Chapter 4)
Assessment, Nursing Diagnosis, and Planning (Chapter 5)

Patient: Piya Jordan, Medical-Surgical Floor, Room 403

Objectives:

- Gather physical and psychosocial information for a database.
- Analyze assessment data to determine patient needs.
- Identify problems and choose appropriate nursing diagnoses for a nursing care plan.
- Prioritize nursing diagnoses for a specific patient.

Nurses use the nursing process continually as they go about their daily duties. Through practice, you will learn to use the nursing process steps in all types of nursing situations. You will use the process for all of your patient assignments—regardless of whether you are caring for a complex patient with a life-threatening illness or assessing the patient who is preparing to undergo a common surgical procedure. Each step of the process is methodical and systematic and requires critical thinking. This lesson will start you on the path to incorporating the nursing process into your practice.

Exercise 1

 CD-ROM Activity—Data Collection

 30 minutes

Assessment requires gathering information about patients and their needs in a variety of ways. Data are systematically obtained and organized into a logical database.

- Sign in to work at Pacific View Regional Hospital on the Medical-Surgical Floor for Period of Care 1. (*Note:* If you are already in the virtual hospital from a previous exercise, click on **Leave the Floor** and then **Restart the Program** to get to the sign-in window.)
- From the Patient List, select Piya Jordan (Room 403).
- Click on **Get Report** and take notes as needed.

1. Review the patient information sheet below and begin recording the data you will need to care for Piya Jordan.

Patient's name: Room: Age:

Allergies:

Diagnoses:

Surgical procedure:

Vital Signs: BP _____ HR _____ RR _____ T _____ SpO$_2$ _____

Pain rating: Last medicated for pain:

Foley: IV:

PCA:

Dressing and drain:

- Click on **Go to Nurses' Station**.
- Click on **Chart** and then on **403**.
- Click on **Physician's Notes** and scroll down to the first note at the bottom to read them in order. Note the diagnosis and general plan.
- Now click on **Return to Nurses' Station** and then on **403** on the bottom toolbar.
- Read the Initial Observation and then click on **Clinical Alerts**.
- Next, click on **Patient Care**.
- Gather physical assessment data by clicking on each of the areas of the body (the yellow boxes) and then on the specific subcategories of that area (the green boxes). Record your findings in question 2 as you progress through the assessment. Remember to click on **Equipment** for each area you assess. (*Hint:* **Equipment** appears in vertical text in the dark green box to the right of the subcategories.)

2.

Assessment Area	Data
Head & Neck Mental Status	
Chest Cardiovascular	
Respiratory	
Abdomen Integumentary	
Upper Extremities Integumentary	
Lower Extremities Musculoskeletal	

3. Consider whether each piece of data below is objective or subjective. Mark with an S for subjective or an O for objective.

_____ a. Has abdominal pain

_____ b. Is confused

_____ c. Pain rated as a "4"

_____ d. Absent bowel sounds

_____ e. Breath sounds clear

_____ f. Restless and agitated

→ • Click on **Chart** and then on **403**.

• Click on the tab for **Nursing Admission** and read the data the nurse recorded during the admission interview. As you read, begin to answer questions 4 through 6.

The physician's History and Physical can provide other relevant data.

→ • Click on the chart tab for **History and Physical**. Review Piya Jordan's History and Physical and take notes as needed to complete questions 4 through 6.

4. What physician's findings are recorded for Piya Jordan's abdominal assessment?

5. For each item listed below and on the next page, record what you have learned based on your review of Piya Jordan's chart.

Religion

Home situation

Alcohol use

Tobacco use

Caffeine use

Previous surgeries

Occupation

Barriers to learning

Best method of instruction

Source of anxiety or fear

6. What is Piya Jordan's family history?

Exercise 2

CD-ROM Activity—Analyzing Data and Determining Problem Areas

30 minutes

Read in your textbook about the signs and symptoms of colon cancer.

1. In the list below, identify the signs and symptoms of colon cancer by marking with an X.

   _____ a. Weakness

   _____ b. Abdominal pain

   _____ c. Weight gain

   _____ d. Nausea and vomiting

   _____ e. Blood in the stool

   _____ f. Dizziness

   _____ g. Change in stool characteristics

• Sign in to work at Pacific View Regional Hospital on the Medical-Surgical Floor for Period of Care 1. (*Note:* If you are already in the virtual hospital from a previous exercise, click on **Leave the Floor** and then **Restart the Program** to get to the sign-in window.)

• From the Patient List, select Piya Jordan (Room 403).

• Click on **Get Report** for Piya Jordan and take notes as needed.

• Click on **Go to Nurses' Station**.

• Click on **Chart** and then on **403**.

• Click on the **Physician's Notes** tab and locate the note concerning the surgical procedure that Piya Jordan underwent.

2. Piya Jordan had a _____.

You have gathered a lot of information in this lesson about Piya Jordan and her condition and problems. Begin to form clusters of the data that are abnormal or indicate a problem.

3. Based on your clusters of data, write three nursing diagnoses in order of priority for Piya Jordan. In parentheses after each nursing diagnosis, include the supporting data.

a.

b.

c.

 • Click on **Return to Nurses' Station**.

• Click on the **Kardex** and then choose **403** for Piya Jordan's Kardex.

• Read through the Kardex, taking notes as needed.

4. Below and on the next page, list the other problem areas for Piya Jordan.

a.

b.

c.

d.

e.

f,

5. Write expected outcomes for the three nursing diagnoses you listed in question 3. (*Hint:* See Chapter 5 in your textbook.)

a.

b.

c.

Applying the Nursing Process: Implementation and Evaluation

📖 **Reading Assignment:** Assessment, Nursing Diagnosis, and Planning (Chapter 5)
Implementation and Evaluation (Chapter 6)
Diet Therapy and Assisted Feeding (Chapter 27)

Patients: Piya Jordan, Medical-Surgical Floor, Room 403
Patricia Newman, Medical-Surgical Floor, Room 406

Objectives:

- Identify appropriate individualized nursing interventions to achieve outcomes.
- Evaluate whether outcomes are being met.

After data were collected and analyzed, problem areas were determined. Then nursing diagnoses were chosen and expected outcomes were written. A plan was formulated to meet those expected outcomes. The next steps in the nursing process are implementation of the plan and evaluation of the actions' results to see whether the expected outcomes have been met. When you have a patient assignment on a hospital unit, you may be given a printout of the care plan. If not, you will need to consult the physician's orders and the Kardex to see just what the nursing orders and the plan of care entail. You will be expected to carry out that plan of care within the limits of your present abilities and knowledge. During your shift you will keep track of data and your actions so that they will be available to determine whether the expected outcomes are being met. You will evaluate the nursing care the patient has received.

Exercise 1

CD-ROM Activity—Choosing Nursing Interventions and Implementing Them

30 minutes

Read about pain and the interventions used to relieve pain on pages 588-589 in your textbook.

- Sign in to work at Pacific View Regional Hospital on the Medical-Surgical Floor for Period of Care 3. (*Note:* If you are already in the virtual hospital from a previous exercise, click on **Leave the Floor** and then **Restart the Program** to get to the sign-in window.)
- From the Patient List, select Piya Jordan (Room 403).
- Click on **Go to Nurses' Station**.
- Click on the **MAR** and then on **403** to review Piya Jordan's medications.

1. What order does Piya Jordan have for pain medication?

→ • Click on **Return to Nurses' Station**. Now access the Drug Guide by clicking on the **Drug** icon in the lower left corner of the screen. Scroll to find meperidine. Read about this medication.

2. What type of pain medication is meperidine?

3. How long does IV meperidine last in the body?
   a. 5 minutes
   b. 1-2 hours
   c. 2-3 hours
   d. 3-4 hours

4. Other than assessing the level of pain the patient is experiencing, what assessment is most important before administering meperidine?
   a. Auscultating bowel sounds
   b. Determining that the patient is alert and oriented
   c. Assessing respirations
   d. Assessing for constipation

→ • Click on **Return to Nurses' Station** and then click on Room **403**.
   • Click on **Take Vital Signs** and record below.

5. Piya Jordan's vital signs at this time are:

   BP _____ SpO$_2$ _____ T _____ HR _____ RR _____ Pain level _____

6. Do you think it is safe for Piya Jordan to be receiving the meperidine via the PCA pump? (*Hint:* See normal values for vital signs on page 343 of your textbook.)

7. Is Piya Jordan's pain well controlled?

8. How would you evaluate whether the expected outcome of pain will be controlled to a level no greater than 3 by medication?

Exercise 2

 CD-ROM Activity—Interventions to Meet Expected Outcomes

 15 minutes

Patricia Newman is receiving medication therapy for a diagnosis of hypertension.

- Sign in to work at Pacific View Regional Hospital on the Medical-Surgical Floor for Period of Care 3. (*Note:* If you are already in the virtual hospital from a previous exercise, click on **Leave the Floor** and then **Restart the Program** to get to the sign-in window.)
- From the Patient List, select Piya Jordan (Room 403) and Patricia Newman (Room 406).
- Click on **Go to Nurses' Station**.
- Click on **MAR** and then on tab **406** to view Patricia Newman's MAR. Scroll down to the second page of the MAR.

1. What is the second medication listed on the second page of the MAR?

 - Click on **Return to Nurses' Station** and then click on the **Drug** icon in the lower left corner of the screen. Scroll to find the medication you identified as the answer to question 1. Read about this drug, which is a beta-adrenergic blocker. The action of this drug is complex—note that it can decrease cardiac output, and yet it is also used to treat decreased cardiac output caused by arrhythmia. Note also that slowing the heart rate decreases the myocardial oxygen demand.

2. What effect does this drug have on the pulse and blood pressure?

3. Which of the following assessments are essential to complete before administering the drug you identified in question 1? Mark your choices with an X.

_____ a. Measure the patient's temperature

_____ b. Measure the apical pulse

_____ c. Measure the blood pressure

_____ d. Assess respirations

_____ e. Check renal function and liver function laboratory results

_____ f. Check the electrolyte laboratory results

_____ g. Auscultate the lungs

Piya Jordan's second nursing diagnosis is Decreased cardiac output. The expected outcome is that the arrhythmia (atrial fibrillation that is causing the decreased cardiac output) will be controlled by medication and diet. Read about arrhythmias and dietary factors that can affect them in your textbook. Pay particular attention to the precautions for the patient with atrial fibrillation.

• Click on **Return to Nurses' Station**; then click on **Chart** and **403** to view Piya Jordan's chart. Click on **Nursing Admission** and read item 10.

4. What does Piya Jordan usually drink?

5. These drinks contain _____, which may make her arrhythmia worse.

6. What dietary restrictions would you suggest to Piya Jordan?

7. How would you evaluate whether the diet restrictions and the medication are effective in meeting the expected outcome of "arrhythmia will be controlled by medication and diet"?

Exercise 3

 CD-ROM Activity—Evaluation

 30 minutes

Another nursing diagnosis for Piya Jordan is Nutrition, risk for less than body requirements. Recall that she has just had a colectomy and has a nasogastric tube connected to low suction. She is NPO. (*Hint:* See the Physician's Orders in the chart.) Care of the tube in the intestinal tract is important with this nursing diagnosis. An expected outcome would be "Patient will not suffer nausea, vomiting, or abdominal distention."

 Read about nasogastric intubation and suction on pages 477-479 in your textbook.

1. Which of the following interventions would you list on Piya Jordan's plan of care? Mark your choice(s) with an X.

   _____ a. Advance the tube ½ inch each day.

   _____ b. Irrigate the tube with 30-60 mL of normal saline each shift.

   _____ c. Check tube placement prior to instilling anything into it.

   _____ d. Verify suction is working and that the tube is extracting stomach secretions.

   _____ e. Disconnect the tube and plug it for an hour each shift.

• Sign in to work at Pacific View Regional Hospital on the Medical-Surgical Floor for Period of Care 3. (*Note:* If you are already in the virtual hospital from a previous exercise, click on **Leave the Floor** and then **Restart the Program** to get to the sign-in window.)
• From the Patient List, select Piya Jordan (Room 403).
• Click on **Go to Nurses' Station**.
• Click on **403** to go to the patient's room.
• Click on **Patient Care** and then on **Physical Assessment**.
• Click on **Abdomen** and then on each subcategory listed in the green boxes.

2. How would you evaluate whether the expected outcome of "Patient will not suffer nausea, vomiting, or abdominal distention" is being met?

3. This expected outcome _____ (is/is not) being met.

4. How would you evaluate whether the expected outcome of "Patient will resume oral feedings by discharge" is being met?

→ • Click on **Chart** and then on **403**.
   • Click on the **Nursing Admission** tab; then scroll to the Nutrition/Metabolic section and read.

5. What shouldn't Piya Jordan have in her diet?

6. What type of food does Piya Jordan prefer?

7. Piya Jordan has lost _____ recently.

This information tells you that a dietary consult is needed for Piya Jordan. Her nutrition will most likely improve after she recovers from surgery and is able to eat again without nausea. Her weight should stabilize then.

LESSON 5

Communication and the Nurse-Patient Relationship

Reading Assignment: Documentation of Nursing Care (Chapter 7)
Communication and the Nurse-Patient Relationship (Chapter 8)

Patients: Clarence Hughes, Medical-Surgical Floor, Room 404
Dorothy Grant, Obstetrics Floor, Room 201

Objectives:

- Identify nurse-patient interactions that are therapeutic.
- Recognize nonverbal communication within the case scenarios.
- Identify techniques to gather further information from patients.
- Document patient care correctly.
- Explain data that should be included when documenting a change in patient condition.

Exercise 1

 CD-ROM Activity—Therapeutic Communication and Empathy

 45 minutes

- Sign in to work at Pacific View Regional Hospital on the Medical-Surgical Floor for Period of Care 1. (*Note:* If you are already in the virtual hospital from a previous exercise, click on **Leave the Floor** and then **Restart the Program** to get to the sign-in window.)
- From the Patient List, select Clarence Hughes (Room 404).
- Click on **Get Report**.
- Read the report and note any data indicating a possible problem.
- Click on **Go to Nurses' Station** and then on **404** to visit the patient's room.
- Click on **Patient Care** and then on **Nurse-Client Interactions**.
- Select and view the video titled **0730: Assessment/Perception of Care**. (*Note:* Check the virtual clock to see whether enough time has elapsed. You can use the fast forward feature to advance the time by two-minute intervals if the video is not yet available. Then click on **Patient Care** and **Nurse-Client Interactions** to refresh the screen.)

1. What nonverbal actions/signs did you observe while watching Clarence Hughes? (*Hint:* See page 101 in your textbook.)

2. Do the nonverbal messages agree with what Clarence Hughes is saying to the nurse?

3. Do you think it is appropriate for the nurse to ask to do the assessment before giving Clarence Hughes the pain medication he is requesting? Why or why not?

 Review the therapeutic communication section on pages 101-106 in your textbook.

4. Was the nurse's first question to Clarence Hughes therapeutic or nontherapeutic? What type of technique did the nurse use by asking this question?

 Read about knee arthroplasty and CPM—continuous passive motion—in your textbook.

5. Is the nurse showing empathy for Clarence Hughes' pain of 8/10 when she says she will put the CPM back on after giving him his pain medication?

6. Which of the following are used when empathy is present? Mark your choice(s) with an X.

_____ a. Reflection of the person's expressed thought

_____ b. Focus on the person's feelings

_____ c. Very close physical proximity

_____ d. Warm tone of voice

_____ e. Suggestions on how to solve the problem

_____ f. A nonjudgmental attitude

➤ • Still in Clarence Hughes' room, click on **Initial Observations** and read the note.
  • Now click on **Clinical Alerts** and read the note.
  • Click on **Take Vital Signs** and record them below.

7. Clarence Hughes' vital signs at this time are:

BP _____ SpO$_2$ _____ T _____ HR _____ RR _____ Pain level _____

➤ • Click on **Patient Care** and then on **Lower Extremities** to obtain a focused assessment on Clarence Hughes. Be sure to click on each of the subcategories in green boxes. (*Note:* Jot down pertinent findings so that you will be able to document the assessment later.)

8. Using your assessment data and the information from the video interactions, write a SOAP note regarding Clarence Hughes' pain and surgical site just as you would for the patient's chart.

S

O

A

P

➤ • Click on **EPR** in the upper right area of the screen. Click on **Login**.
  • In the Patient box in the upper left area of the screen, select **404** from the drop-down menu. Verify that this is the EPR for Clarence Hughes. Keep **Vital Signs** as the category.
  • In the correct column, enter the vital signs and pain assessment data you obtained above. Highlight each pertinent line to view the codes and meanings available to you.
  • Click on **Exit EPR** and then on **Chart**. Click on the chart for **404** and select **Nurse's Notes**.
  • Read the nurse's note relevant to the 0730 nurse-client interaction you observed.

9. What type of documentation did the nurse use to write this nurse's note? Mark your choice with an X.

_____ a. POMR

_____ b. DAR

_____ c. PIE

_____ d. Focus charting

_____ e. Narrative charting

_____ f. Charting by exception

10. Is the information obtained from the patient about his pain subjective or objective data?

Exercise 2

CD-ROM Activity—More Therapeutic Techniques

15 minutes

- Sign in to work at Pacific View Regional Hospital on the Obstetrics Floor for Period of Care 2. (*Note:* If you are already in the virtual hospital from a previous exercise, click on **Leave the Floor** and then **Restart the Program** to get to the sign-in window.)
- From the Patient List, select Dorothy Grant (Room 201).
- Click on **Get Report** and read the report. Note that Dorothy Grant was admitted after domestic abuse by her husband. She is experiencing early labor. She is frightened for herself and her children.
- Click on **Go to Nurses' Station** and then on **201** at the bottom of the screen.
- Click on **Patient Care** and then on **Nurse-Client Interactions**.
- Select and view the video titled **1115: Nurse-Patient Communication**. (*Note:* Check the virtual clock to see whether enough time has elapsed. You can use the fast forward feature to advance the time by two-minute intervals if the video is not yet available. Then click on **Patient Care** and **Nurse-Client Interactions** to refresh the screen.)

1. What nonverbal communication does the nurse use at the start of the interaction?

2. What does the nurse say to open the interaction?

3. What type of technique was the beginning statement made by the nurse? (*Hint:* See Table 8-1 in your textbook.)

   _____ a. General lead

   _____ b. Reflection

   _____ c. Seeking clarification

   _____ d. Focusing

   _____ e. Encouraging elaboration

4. Dorothy states that she is scared, and the nurse responds with _____

   _____.

5. This statement by the nurse is an example of which therapeutic technique?

6. The nurse states that the social worker and the nurse specialist will work together to identify Dorothy Grant's immediate needs. What is this communication technique used by the nurse called?

7. Did you find any blocks to effective communication in this interaction?

8. The nurse was _____ (empathetic/nonempathetic) in this interaction.

LESSON 6

Documentation of Nursing Care

Reading Assignment: Documentation of Nursing Care (Chapter 7)

Patients: Clarence Hughes, Medical-Surgical Floor, Room 404
Harry George, Medical-Surgical Floor, Room 401

Objectives:

- Document patient care in electronic patient records.
- Identify data that should be documented in the nurse's notes.
- Correctly document in the nurse's notes.
- List data that should be included when documenting a change in condition.

Since the patient's record is a legal document, it is essential to learn to document correctly and completely. Always become familiar with the official charting format required at the clinical facility to which you are assigned. Documentation styles vary considerably from one facility to another. Documentation is done in several different sections of a chart and on the Kardex or electronic care plan. In this lesson you will familiarize yourself with the documentation areas of the chart using a particular scenario, noting what is recorded in the Electronic Patient Record (EPR), on the Medication Administration Record (MAR), the Kardex, the Nurse's Notes, Physician's Progress Notes, and Consultations.

Exercise 1

 CD-ROM Activity—Exploring Documentation

 45 minutes

- Sign in to work at Pacific View Regional Hospital on the Medical-Surgical Floor for Period of Care 2. (*Note:* If you are already in the virtual hospital from a previous exercise, click on **Leave the Floor** and then **Restart the Program** to get to the sign-in window.)
- From the Patient List, select Clarence Hughes (Room 404).
- Click on **Get Report** and review.
- Click on **Go to Nurses' Station** and then click on Room **404**.
- Inside the patient's room, click on **Take Vital Signs**.

77

1. Clarence Hughes' current vital signs are:

BP _____ SpO$_2$ _____ T _____ HR _____ RR _____ Pain level _____

→ • Read the Initial Observation.

• Click on **Clinical Alerts** and read the note.

• Click on **Patient Care** and then on **Nurse-Client Interactions**.

• Select and view the video titled **1115: Interventions—Airway**. (*Note*: Check the virtual clock to see whether enough time has elapsed. You can use the fast forward feature to advance the time by two-minute intervals if the video is not yet available. Then click on **Patient Care** and **Nurse-Client Interactions** to refresh the screen.)

• Now click on **Patient Care** and then on **Chest**.

• Click on each subcategory for the chest assessment and note any abnormal data.

• Click on **EPR** and then on **Login**. Select **404** in the Patient box; keep **Vital Signs** as the category. Verify that this is the EPR for Clarence Hughes.

• In the correct column, enter the vital sign data you obtained in question 1.

• Now change the category to **Respiratory**. Enter the data you obtained during that portion of the chest assessment. Highlight each line to see the codes and meanings you may use for that specific item.

• Next, choose the **Cardiovascular** category and enter that assessment data.

• Finally, change the category to **Psychosocial** and enter the data regarding Clarence Hughes' anxiety.

• Return to the **Vital Signs** category.

2. Which vital sign measurements have changed considerably since they were last taken? Mark your choices with an X.

_____ a. Blood pressure

_____ b. Temperature

_____ c. Heart rate

_____ d. SpO$_2$

_____ e. Respiratory rate

3. What nonverbal communication did you observe in the nurse-client video interaction that indicated Clarence Hughes is in distress?

4. Using a focus charting format, write a nurse's note regarding the change in Clarence Hughes' condition. (*Hint:* See page 87 in your textbook.)

D

A

R

 • Before leaving the EPR, familiarize yourself with the various available charting sections of this electronic format by choosing each category in turn and looking at the data lines available for that area.

• Now click on **Exit EPR** and then on **Chart**. Select **404** and click on **Nurse's Notes**.

• Compare the nurse's note in the chart with the note you wrote for question 4.

5. Did you leave anything important out of the nurse's note you wrote for question 4?

Exercise 2

 CD-ROM Activity—Documentation Practice

 45 minutes

• Sign in to work at Pacific View Regional Hospital on the Medical-Surgical Floor for Period of Care 1. (*Note:* If you are already in the virtual hospital from a previous exercise, click on **Leave the Floor** and then **Restart the Program** to get to the sign-in window.)

• From the Patient List, select Harry George (Room 401).

• Click on **Get Report** and read the report.

• Click on **Go to Nurses' Station** and then on **401** to go to Harry George's room.

• Read the Initial Observation.

• Click on **Clinical Alerts** to determine whether there is an immediate nursing need.

• Click on **Take Vital Signs**.

1. Harry George's vital signs are:

BP _____ SpO$_2$ _____ T _____ HR _____ RR _____ Pain level _____

• Perform a brief assessment on Harry George.
  • First, click on **Patient Care** and then click on **Physical Assessment**.
  • Click on **Head & Neck** and then select **Mental Status** from the green boxes.

  2. What is Harry George's current mental status?

 • Click on **Lower Extremities** and then click on each of the available subcategories.
  • Make note below of any pertinent findings for later entry in the EPR or Nurse's Notes.

  3. What do your findings from the assessment of Harry George's lower extremities reveal?

→ • Click on **EPR** in the right corner of the screen and then click **Login**.
  • Select **401** in the Patient box. Verify that you are in Harry George's EPR.
  • With **Vital Signs** in the Category box, locate the Wed 0730 time column. Record your vital signs findings from question 1.
  • Using the Category drop-down menu, choose **Cardiovascular** and enter the data you obtained from the vascular assessment of the lower extremities.
  • Now change the Category to **Neurologic** and enter the data you obtained regarding Harry George's mental status.
  • Change the Category to **Musculoskeletal** and enter the data you obtained when you assessed the lower extremities.
  • Next, select **Integumentary** as the Category and enter the appropriate code for the assessment of the lower extremities.
  • Finally, select the Category of **Wounds and Drains** and enter the codes for the assessment of Harry George's leg wound.

4. Now write a nurse's note for the remaining assessment data that you could not record in the EPR. Use source-oriented or narrative charting. (*Hint:* See pages 83-84 in your textbook.)

 • Click on **Exit EPR**.
   • Click on **Chart** and then **401**.
   • Click on the **Physician's Orders** tab.
   • Find the order for pain medication.

   5. The medication ordered for Harry George's pain is _____

   _____.

 • Click on **Return to Room 401** and then on **MAR**. Select tab **401** and search for the pain medication written in the physician's order.

   6. Harry George received the new pain medication at _____.

 • Click on **Return to Room 401**.
   • Click on **Chart** and then **401**.
   • Click on the **Nurse's Notes** tab and read the note for the beginning of this shift.

   7. What does the nurse's note say about Harry George's pain level and administration of pain medication?

Exercise 3

 CD-ROM Activity—Other Charting Formats

 30 minutes

   • Sign in to work at Pacific View Regional Hospital on the Medical-Surgical Floor for Period of Care 1. (*Note:* If you are already in the virtual hospital from a previous exercise, click on **Leave the Floor** and then **Restart the Program** to get to the sign-in window.)
   • From the Patient List, select Harry George (Room 401).
   • Click on **Go to Nurses' Station**.

1. Data obtained from the patient verbally are called subjective data. Data obtained by hands-on physical assessment or through the senses are objective data. Consider whether each piece of data below is objective or subjective. Mark with an S for subjective or an O for objective.

   _____ a. "My pain is at 8/10."

   _____ b. Left lower leg erythematous from toes to mid-calf.

   _____ c. "It hurts to move my foot."

   _____ d. Serous drainage from wound.

   _____ e. Temperature 100.2 degrees F.

   _____ f. "Bring me my bottle and a cigarette."

2. Match each piece of assessment data listed below with the location in the patient record where it should be documented.

   Data Obtained

   _____ Open lesion 2-3 cm on left ankle

   _____ Right pedal pulse 2+

   _____ Pain at 6/10

   _____ Skin erythematous from toes to mid-calf of left leg

   _____ Impaired ROM in left leg

   _____ Asking for alcohol and cigarettes

   _____ Alert and oriented to person, place, and situation

   _____ Hydromorphone 2 mg IV given at 0715

   Where to Document Data

   a. Chart only

   b. EPR only

   c. Chart and EPR

3. The charting by exception format assumes that _____ unless documented to the contrary. (*Hint:* See page 89 in your textbook.)
   a. the body system was assessed
   b. data obtained are irrelevant
   c. all standards and protocols were followed
   d. a full physical assessment has been performed

4. Which of the following are true of the charting guidelines for correct, legally accurate documentation? Mark your choices with an X. (*Hint:* See pages 92-95 in your textbook.)

_____ a. Use only agency-accepted symbols and abbreviations in documentation.

_____ b. Visitors should be mentioned by name.

_____ c. Physician visits should be documented.

_____ d. Start each sentence with a capital letter and end with a period.

_____ e. Use complete sentences when documenting in the nurse's notes.

_____ f. When the patient is the subject of the sentence, leave "patient" out of the sentence.

_____ g. Do not duplicate the charting of an item on a flow sheet in the nurse's notes.

_____ h. Chart only what you have performed or observed.

_____ i. Pencil may be used on a flow sheet.

_____ j. Entries must not be erased or covered with any type of correction fluid.

• Click on **401** to go to the patient's room.
• Click on **Patient Care** and then on **Nurse-Client Interactions**.
• Select and view the video titled **0810: The Patient in Pain**. (*Note:* Check the virtual clock to see whether enough time has elapsed. You can use the fast forward feature to advance the time by two-minute intervals if the video is not yet available. Then click on **Patient Care** and **Nurse-Client Interactions** to refresh the screen.)

5. Write a SOAP note regarding the interaction you just observed. (*Hint:* Review the SOAP format on pages 85-86 of your textbook.)

S

O

A

P

6. PIE charting is another style of charting. Document the nurse-client interaction you observed using the PIE format.

P

I

E

Psychosocial Concerns

Reading Assignment: Concepts of Health, Illness, and Health Promotion (Chapter 2)
Adulthood and the Family (Chapter 12)
Loss, Grief, and the Dying Patient (Chapter 15)
Common Psychosocial Care Problems of the Elderly
(Chapter 41)

Patients: Kathryn Doyle, Skilled Nursing Floor, Room 503
Harry George, Medical-Surgical Floor, Room 401

Objectives:

- Gather psychosocial data about the patient for the database.
- Identify specific stresses caused by surgery, an illness, and/or hospitalization.
- Describe the types of losses experienced by patient in the case scenario.

Psychosocial care of the patient is very important and should not be overlooked in the process of giving physical care. Each patient is a unique individual with personal concerns related to his or her state of health or illness. Hospitalization disrupts roles and creates stress for the patient and the family. Some psychosocial data are available from the patient's chart. Eliciting further data is usually done after the nurse has established some rapport with the patient. Most patients appreciate it when the nurse knows a little about what they do outside of the hospital, what family members they have, and whether or not spirituality is important in their life. Finding out about the patient by reading the chart before your first meeting provides information that you can use to open conversation and gain insight into your patient's unique life situation. For instance, just knowing whether the patient has health insurance can provide an idea of how much financial stress is caused by hospitalization. An initial idea about the patient's support systems can also be derived from chart information. Is the patient married? What ages are the patient's children? Is this patient active in a church, other spiritual group, or a community organization? For all these reasons, it is good practice to perform a chart review *before* beginning patient care.

Exercise 1

 CD-ROM Activity—Psychosocial Assessment

30 minutes

- Sign in to work at Pacific View Regional Hospital on the Skilled Nursing Floor for Period of Care 1. (*Note:* If you are already in the virtual hospital from a previous exercise, click on **Leave the Floor** and then **Restart the Program** to get to the sign-in window.)
- From the Patient List, select Kathryn Doyle (Room 503).
- Click on **Get Report**.
- Click on **Go to Nurses' Station**.
- Click on **Chart** and then on **503**; verify that this is the chart for Kathryn Doyle.
- Review the **Admissions** and the **Nursing Admissions** sections of the chart.

1. Fill in the form below based on your review of Kathryn Doyle's chart.

Age:	Marital status:	Children:
Religion or spiritual base:		Actively involved?
Health insurance:		Employment:
Language spoken:		Educational level:
Previous hospitalization:		
Stress factors:		
Self-perception:		
Fears:		

2. What surgical procedure did Kathryn Doyle undergo? (*Hint:* Read about this procedure in your medical-surgical textbook.)

3. This procedure has an impact on self-concept for many women. From reading the Nursing Admission, do you think this surgery will have an impact on Kathryn Doyle's self-concept? Explain your answer.

- Click on **Return to Nurses' Station**.
- Click on **503** to go to the patient's room.
- Inside the room, click on **Patient Care** and then on **Nurse-Client Interactions**.
- Select and review the video titled **0730: Assessment—Biophysical**. (*Note:* Check the virtual clock to see whether enough time has elapsed. You can use the fast forward feature to advance the time by two-minute intervals if the video is not yet available. Then click on **Patient Care** and **Nurse-Client Interactions** to refresh the screen.)

4. During this video interaction, what concern does the nurse discover that Kathryn Doyle has?

- Once again, click on **Patient Care** and then on **Nurse-Client Interactions**.
- To answer question 5, you will need to select and view two more nurse-client interaction videos: **0733: Planning—Fact Finding** and **0740: Planning for Care**. (*Note:* Check the virtual clock to see whether enough time has elapsed. You can use the fast forward feature to advance the time by two-minute intervals if the video is not yet available. Then click on **Patient Care** and **Nurse-Client Interactions** to refresh the screen.)

5. The second and third interactions give data about Kathryn Doyle's nutritional status. What stressors were identified?

Exercise 2

 CD-ROM Activity—An Added Stressor

 30 minutes

- Sign in to work at Pacific View Regional Hospital on the Skilled Nursing Floor for Period of Care 2. (*Note:* If you are already in the virtual hospital from a previous exercise, click on **Leave the Floor** and then **Restart the Program** to get to the sign-in window.)
- From the Patient List, select Kathryn Doyle (Room 503).
- Click on **Get Report** and read the note.
- Click on **Go to Nurses' Station** and then on **503**.
- Inside the patient's room, click on **Patient Care** and then on **Nurse-Client Interactions**.
- Select and view the video titled **1115: An Unexpected Visitor**. (*Note*: Check the virtual clock to see whether enough time has elapsed. You can use the fast forward feature to advance the time by two-minute intervals if the video is not yet available. Then click on **Patient Care** and **Nurse-Client Interactions** to refresh the screen.)

1. Who is visiting Kathryn Doyle?

 - Once again, click on **Patient Care** and then on **Nurse-Client Interactions**.
- Now select and view the video titled **1120: ORIF—Physical Therapy**. (*Note*: Check the virtual clock to see whether enough time has elapsed. You can use the fast forward feature to advance the time by two-minute intervals if the video is not yet available. Then click on **Patient Care** and **Nurse-Client Interactions** to refresh the screen.)

2. What does Kathryn Doyle ask the nurse?

3. Kathryn Doyle asks Trevor to go with her to physical therapy. How does he reply?

- The physician ordered a consult by the psychiatric nurse specialist to assess Kathryn Doyle.
- Click on **Chart** and then on **503**; select the chart tab for **Consultations**.
- Read the Psychiatric Nurse Specialist Consult.

4. What other concerns did this psychiatric nurse specialist identify? (*Hint:* See the Findings section of the consult.)

5. What conclusions did the nurse come to about Kathryn Doyle? (*Hint:* See Impressions in the consult.)

→ • Click on **Return to Room 503**.
   • Click on **Patient Care** and then on **Nurse-Client Interactions**.
   • Select and view the video titled **1130: The Unexpected Event**. (*Note*: Check the virtual clock to see whether enough time has elapsed. You can use the fast forward feature to advance the time by two-minute intervals if the video is not yet available. Then click on **Patient Care** and **Nurse-Client Interactions** to refresh the screen.)

6. What did you observe Trevor do?

7. What did Trevor say when the nurse walked in and asked him what he was doing?

Read about crimes against the elderly on pages 830-832 in your textbook.

8. There are several categories of elder abuse. What type of elder abuse do you consider Trevor's action? Mark your choice with an X.

_____ a. Physical abuse

_____ b. Sexual abuse

_____ c. Psychological abuse

_____ d. Material abuse

_____ e. Neglect

9. Considering that she has lost 10 pounds since she moved into her son's home, Kathryn

Doyle's son not taking her to the dentist could constitute _____.

10. How will these issues be dealt with? What is the plan of the psychiatric nurse specialist?

 11. Considering what you have learned about Kathryn Doyle and her stress so far, name four measures that might help decrease her stress and anxiety while she is in the hospital. (*Hint:* See Table 2-6 on page 23 of your textbook.)

12. It has just been discovered that Trevor has stolen money from Kathryn Doyle. Considering the psychosocial history that the patient has reported regarding how her son has taken over her life and finances, for which of the following crimes against the elderly should an assessment be made?
   a. Assault
   b. Fraudulent schemes
   c. Investment fraud
   d. Medical quackery

Exercise 3

 CD-ROM Activity—Homelessness

 30 minutes

- Sign in to work at Pacific View Regional Hospital on the Medical-Surgical Floor for Period of Care 3. (*Note:* If you are already in the virtual hospital from a previous exercise, click on **Leave the Floor** and then **Restart the Program** to get to the sign-in window.)
- From the Patient List, select Harry George (Room 401).
- Click on **Get Report** and read.

1. What psychosocial concerns does Harry George have according to the report?

➤ • Click on **Go to Nurses' Station** and then on Room **401**.
  • Read the Initial Observation.

2. What psychosocial activity is occurring at this time?

➤ • Click on **Chart** and select the **Nursing Admission** tab. Review as needed to complete question 3.

3. Fill in the information below from the Nursing Admission.

Self-Perception

Role Relationships

Coping and Stress Tolerance

Life Principles

→ • Click on the **Consultations** tab of the chart and read the Psychiatric Consult.

4. The two major psychiatric problems identified are _____ and

_____.

5. How do you think Harry George's underlying physical problems are a factor in his psychiatric problems?

6. The psychiatric nurse consultant recommends that Harry George be started on

_____.

7. Which of the following did the psychiatric nurse consultant recommend? Mark your choices with an X.

_____ a. In-patient psychiatric hospitalization

_____ b. Affiliation with alcoholics anonymous

_____ c. Enrollment in vocational rehabilitation and skills training

_____ d. Group therapy for alcohol addiction

_____ e. Social service support for finding housing

_____ f. Social service support for continued psychiatric care

_____ g. Social service support for continued medical care

_____ h. Cognitive behavioral therapy for depression

LESSON 8

Loss, Grief, and the Dying Patient

 Reading Assignment: Cultural and Spiritual Aspects of Patient Care (Chapter 14)

Loss, Grief, and the Dying Patient (Chapter 15)

Patient: Goro Oishi, Skilled Nursing Floor, Room 505

Objectives:

- Describe the grief reactions experienced by people in the case scenario.
- Identify ways to meet the spiritual needs of patients in the case scenario.
- Recognize cultural differences in the way death is perceived.

Exercise 1

 CD-ROM Activity—Advance Directives

30 minutes

- Sign in to work at Pacific View Regional Hospital on the Skilled Nursing Floor for Period of Care 1. (*Note:* If you are already in the virtual hospital from a previous exercise, click on **Leave the Floor** and then **Restart the Program** to get to the sign-in window.)
- From the Patient List, select Goro Oishi (Room 505).
- Click on **Get Report** and read the note.
- Click on **Go to Nurses' Station**.
- Click on **Chart** and then on **505**.
- Choose the **Physician's Orders** tab and read the orders.
- Click on the tab for **Admissions** and read through the information.

1. Does Goro Oishi have an advance directive?

2. Which of the following are usually present in hospice care? Mark your choices with an X. (*Hint:* See pages 185-186 in your textbook.)

_____ a. Focus on symptom management

_____ b. Focus on comfort care

_____ c. Care for the family

_____ d. Rigorous treatment of infection

_____ e. Rigorous invasive measures to prolong life

_____ f. Care in the hospital, home, or other facility

3. The type of care delivered within a hospice program is often termed

_____.

4. Considering Goro Oishi's condition, his advance directive, and the principles of hospice/palliative care, which of the following nursing actions would be appropriate for him this shift? Mark your choices with an X. (*Hint:* See pages 188-190 in your textbook and the Physician's Orders for today.)

_____ a. Instill lubricating eye drops

_____ b. Prepare to insert feeding tube

_____ c. Assess IV site every 2 hours

_____ d. Monitor oxygen saturation

_____ e. Monitor urine output via Foley catheter

_____ f. Medicate for nausea

_____ g. Turn and reposition every 2 hours

_____ h. Assess skin for pressure areas every 2 hours

_____ i. Medicate for elevated temperature

_____ j. Get him up to the chair once a shift

_____ k. Talk to him as care is provided

_____ l. Give him a bed bath

_____ m. Seek an order for constipation

_____ n. Provide urinary catheter care

• Click on **Return to Nurses' Station** and then on **505** to go to the patient's room.

  • Inside the room, click on **Patient Care** and then on **Nurse-Client Interactions**.

  • Select and view the video titled **0735: Assessment—Family**. (*Note*: Check the virtual clock to see whether enough time has elapsed. You can use the fast forward feature to advance the time by two-minute intervals if the video is not yet available. Then click on **Patient Care** and **Nurse-Client Interactions** to refresh the screen.)

5. What do you think Mrs. Oishi means when she tells the nurse that she wishes her son would accept his father's wishes?

6. The interaction indicates that this son is _____ to let his father go.

 • Again, click on **Patient Care** and then on **Nurse-Client Interactions**.

  • To complete the remaining questions in this exercise, you need to view two more nurse-client video interactions: **0745: Intervention—Clarification** and **0750: Family Conflict—Plan of Care**. (*Note*: Check the virtual clock to see whether enough time has elapsed. You can use the fast forward feature to advance the time by two-minute intervals if the video is not yet available. Then click on **Patient Care** and **Nurse-Client Interactions** to refresh the screen.)

There are several stages of grief. Various family members may go through different phases at different times. Hospice nurses are familiar with this and can tactfully deal with each family member. It is too early to really assess the grief reaction of each member of the Oishi family, but you can determine the initial reaction of each family member.

7. Match each family member with his or her present stage of grief.

Family Member	**Stage of Grief**
_____ Mrs. Oishi (patient's wife)	a. Shock and disbelief
_____ Kiyoshi (youngest son)	b. Protest
_____ Namishi (oldest son)	c. Disorganization
	d. Reorganization

 8. An advance directive (*Hint:* See page 191 in your textbook.)
  a. states the patient's wishes in case of illness.
  b. spells out the patient's wishes for health care when patient is unable to indicate his or her choice.
  c. legally appoints a person to carry out one's wishes.
  d. is aimed at prolonging life.

9. What are three advantages of having an advance directive in place?

Exercise 2

 CD-ROM Activity—Signs of Deterioration

 30 minutes

In addition to an advance directive, a patient may have a signed durable power of attorney. Mrs. Oishi has the durable power of attorney for health care for Goro Oishi.

- Sign in to work at Pacific View Regional Hospital on the Skilled Nursing Floor for Period of Care 2. (*Note:* If you are already in the virtual hospital from a previous exercise, click on **Leave the Floor** and then **Restart the Program** to get to the sign-in window.)
- From the Patient List, select Goro Oishi (Room 505).
- Click on **Get Report** and read the report.
- Click on **Go to Nurses' Station**.
- Click on **505** and then on **Take Vital Signs**.

  1. Goro Oishi's current vital signs are:

  BP _____ SpO$_2$ _____ T _____ HR _____ RR _____

 - Click on and read the **Initial Observations** and the **Clinical Alerts**.
- Click on **EPR** and then on **Login**. Select **505** from the Patient drop-down menu. Keep **Vital Signs** in the Category box.
- Enter Goro Oishi's vital signs in the appropriate time column.
- Scroll back using the arrow at the bottom of the screen to compare the vital signs from previous times.

  2. Complete the table below by entering the vital signs from the EPR for the days and times specified.

Assessment of Vital Sign Trends

	Tues 0600	Tues 1400	Wed 1129
Blood pressure			
SpO$_2$			
Temperature			
Heart rate			
Respiratory rate			

3. What changes or trends do you see in the vital signs?

BP

SpO$_2$

T

HR

RR

4. Which of the following are physical signs of approaching death? Mark your choices with an X. (*Hint:* See page 190 in your textbook.)

_____ a. Temperature rises

_____ b. Heart rate rises

_____ c. Heart rate drops

_____ d. Blood pressure rises

_____ e. Blood pressure drops

_____ f. Respirations become irregular

_____ g. Extremities become mottled, cool, and dusky

• Click on **Exit EPR** to return to Room 505.

• Click on **Patient Care** and then on **Nurse-Client Interactions**.

• Select and view the video titled **1117: Spiritual Beliefs—Death, Dying**. (*Note:* Check the virtual clock to see whether enough time has elapsed. You can use the fast forward feature to advance the time by two-minute intervals if the video is not yet available. Then click on **Patient Care** and **Nurse-Client Interactions** to refresh the screen.)

5. Goro Oishi's religion is _____.

6. Considering the fact that Goro Oishi is comatose and unresponsive, it is impossible for the family to interact with him. What should the nurse caution the family to be careful about when in Goro Oishi's room? (*Hint:* See page 190 in your textbook.)

• Once again, click on **Patient Care** and then on **Nurse-Client Interactions**.

• Now select and view the video titled **1125: The Family Facing Death**. (*Note:* Check the virtual clock to see whether enough time has elapsed. You can use the fast forward feature to advance the time by two-minute intervals if the video is not yet available. Then click on **Patient Care** and **Nurse-Client Interactions** to refresh the screen.)

7. Who is present here besides the family?

8. Does the younger son seem open to hearing any discussion of Goro Oishi's beliefs?

9. What does the nurse tell the family?

10. What is the younger son's response?

➡ • Click on **Patient Care** and then **Nurse-Client Interactions**.
   • Select and view the video titled **1126: The Medical Power of Attorney**. (*Note*: Check the virtual clock to see whether enough time has elapsed. You can use the fast forward feature to advance the time by two-minute intervals if the video is not yet available. Then click on **Patient Care** and **Nurse-Client Interactions** to refresh the screen.)

11. Which of the following does Mrs. Oishi try to explain to her son?

_____ a. She was chosen by her husband as his "agent" in case he reached the end of his life.

_____ b. She loves her husband and wants him to live.

_____ c. She wishes to respect his (Goro Oishi's) wishes.

_____ d. She wishes to allow her husband to die with dignity.

_____ e. There is no way that her husband's condition will allow him to live.

Exercise 3

 CD-ROM Activity—Signs of Impending Death

 15 minutes

- Sign in to work at Pacific View Regional Hospital on the Skilled Nursing Floor for Period of Care 3. (*Note:* If you are already in the virtual hospital from a previous exercise, click on **Leave the Floor** and then **Restart the Program** to get to the sign-in window.)
- From the Patient List, select Goro Oishi (Room 505).
- Click on **Get Report** and read the note.
- Click on **Go to Nurses' Station** and then on **505** to go to the patient's room.
- Read the Initial Observation.

1. Among the changes in Goro Oishi's condition, his left eye has become

   _____.

2. A change noted in the Initial Observation that indicates Goro Oishi's kidneys have shut

   down is _____ for the last 4 hours.

 • Click on **Take Vital Signs**.

3. Goro Oishi's current vital signs are:

BP_____ SpO$_2$ _____ T _____ HR _____ RR _____

4. Compare these current vital signs with the last ones you measured. What changes do you see in the vital signs now?

• Click on **Patient Care** and then on **Nurse-Client Interactions**.
- Select and view the video titled **1500: Patient Decline**. (*Note:* Check the virtual clock to see whether enough time has elapsed. You can use the fast forward feature to advance the time by two-minute intervals if the video is not yet available. Then click on **Patient Care** and **Nurse-Client Interactions** to refresh the screen.)
- Click again on **Patient Care** and then on **Nurse-Client Interactions**.
- Next, select and view the video titled **1505: Meeting the Spiritual Needs**.

5. What change is happening to Goro Oishi?

6. The family requests that _____ be called.

Goro Oishi's vital signs cease and the nurse calls the physician.

7. After Goro Oishi's vital signs cease, the nurse should do which of the following? Mark your choices with an X. (*Hint:* See page 192 of your textbook.)

_____ a. Ask the family members whether they wish to help prepare the body.

_____ b. Allow the family time alone with the patient.

_____ c. Remove tubes and cleanse the body.

_____ d. Prepare the body for the mortuary or coroner.

_____ e. Ask whether the family wants the nurse to stay with them while they view the body.

_____ f. Offer condolences.

Vital Signs, Health Status Assessment, and Data Collection

⌾🕮 **Reading Assignment:** Measuring Vital Signs (Chapter 21)
Assessing Health Status (Chapter 22)

Patients: Pablo Rodriguez, Medical-Surgical Floor, Room 405
Patricia Newman, Medical-Surgical Floor, Room 406

Objectives:

- Recognize abnormal vital signs.
- Identify abnormal findings from the physical assessment.
- Identify priority areas of assessment for specific patients.
- Determine components needed for a focused assessment for identified actual or potential problems.

Accurately measuring vital signs is a basic nursing skill that you will use with every patient. Identifying and interpreting vital sign trends is essential in order to identify complications or problems early. Often it is a subtle change in vital signs that will alert you to perform a thorough physical assessment. Data gathered may help identify the specific systemic change that is causing the vital sign changes or abnormalities. When you can alert the physician to changes in patient physical status, early intervention can often rectify the problem before it becomes serious. The findings you obtain will help the physician determine the most appropriate medical therapies.

Careful physical assessment and data collection provide the information necessary to determine patient needs and the type of nursing interventions that are required to assist the patient in alleviating problems. After interventions have been carried out, vital sign measurement and physical assessment provide the evaluation data to determine that interventions have been successful in meeting the expected outcomes. Data obtained also assist in helping you set priorities for care. For example, if the patient's blood pressure is rising considerably above normal on each successive measurement, you would need to obtain treatment for the hypertension. This would be a higher priority than bathing or ambulating the patient. If a patient's temperature showed an upward trend, you would need to examine the patient for other signs of infection so that proper treatment could be instituted. This would take priority over attending to activity needs.

Exercise 1

 CD-ROM Activity—Normal Versus Abnormal Vital Signs

 45 minutes

Observing trends in vital signs often gives clues to patient problems.

- Sign in to work at Pacific View Regional Hospital on the Medical-Surgical Floor for Period of Care 3. (*Note:* If you are already in the virtual hospital from a previous exercise, click on **Leave the Floor** and then **Restart the Program** to get to the sign-in window.)
- From the Patient List, select Pablo Rodriguez (Room 405).
- Click on **Get Report** and read the note.
- Click on **Go to Nurses' Station**.
- Click on Room **405** and then on **Take Vital Signs**. Record your findings in the bottom row of the table below question 1.
- Click on **EPR** and then on **Login**. Choose **405** in the Patient box. Keep **Vital Signs** in the Category box. Verify that the page you are on is for Pablo Rodriguez.
- Use the blue backward arrow at the bottom of the screen to scroll to the previous vital sign recordings.

  1. In the top three rows of the table below, enter Pablo Rodriguez's earlier vital signs from the EPR. Based on these data and your current findings, begin to analyze the trend of each vital sign.

Day	Time	BP	SpO$_2$	T	HR	RR	Pain
Wed							
Wed							
Wed							
Current findings							

  2. From your analysis of the vital sign trends, what do you think is causing the changes in Pablo Rodriguez's heart rate and respiration?

  3. The normal adult range for temperature is _____. The

     normal pulse range for an adult is _____. The normal range for respira-

     tions in the healthy adult is _____. The normal blood pressure for the

     adult is _____.

4. Imagine you are applying the cuff of a manual sphygmomanometer to a patient's arm. From the list below, choose the appropriate steps for this procedure and number them in the correct order (from 1 to 4). You will not use all the steps listed. (*Hint:* For more information, refer to pages 348-349 in your textbook.)

_____   Place the cuff ½ inch above the antecubital space.

_____   Center the bladder over the brachial artery.

_____   Verify that the cuff is 1½ times the diameter of the patient's arm.

_____   Wrap the cuff smoothly but securely around the arm.

_____   Place the cuff 1 to 2 inches above the antecubital space.

_____   Obtain a cuff that is 21% larger than the patient's arm.

5. When measuring the patient's respirations, what is the rationale for telling the patient you are measuring the pulse when you are really checking respirations?

6. In the list below, place an X by each choice that correctly finishes the following statement. Taking an oral temperature would be contraindicated in a patient who:

_____   a. Has been running a high temperature.

_____   b. Has had previous seizures.

_____   c. Has just finished breakfast.

_____   d. Is 7 years old.

_____   e. Suffers from dementia.

_____   f. Finished a cold soft drink 15 minutes ago.

_____   g. Is newly postoperative.

_____   h. Is a teenager with a leg fracture.

_____   i. Is 2½ years old.

7. A rectal temperature is:
   a. 1 degree higher than an oral temperature.
   b. 1 degree lower than an oral temperature.

Exercise 2

 CD-ROM Activity—Assessment and Data Collection

 45 minutes

Pablo Rodriguez has advanced cancer of the lung. He has received 6 months of chemotherapy followed by irradiation treatment. He was admitted complaining of nausea, vomiting, and increased pain. Perform a focused assessment at this time, evaluating his respiratory and gastrointestinal status.

• Sign in to work at Pacific View Regional Hospital on the Medical-Surgical Floor for Period of Care 3. (*Note:* If you are already in the virtual hospital from a previous exercise, click on **Leave the Floor** and then **Restart the Program** to get to the sign-in window.)
• From the Patient List, select Pablo Rodriguez (Room 405).
• Click on **Go to Nurses' Station**.
• Click on **405** to go to the patient's room.
• Inside the room, click on **Patient Care** and then on **Physical Assessment**.
• Click on **Chest** and then on each assessment subcategory in turn. Note the findings below.
• Click on **Abdomen** and then on each assessment subcategory in turn. Note the findings below.

1. Below, record your findings from the focused assessment of Pablo Rodriguez.

Focused Assessment

Chest
  Integumentary

  Cardiovascular

  Respiratory

  Musculoskeletal

Abdomen
  Integumentary

  Musculoskeletal

  Gastrointestinal

2. On the diagram below, indicate where you should place your stethoscope to properly listen to the lung sounds. (*Hint:* Review lung assessment in your textbook on pages 364-365.)

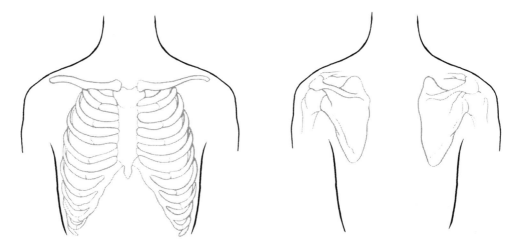

 • Click on **Chart** and then on **405**.
   • Select **Nurse's Notes** and read through the notes.

3. Note indications of problems that should be considered when writing Pablo Rodriguez's care plan.

4. Which of the following would be appropriate nursing diagnoses, considering the data you have gathered from your physical assessment and the chart? Mark your choices with an X.

_____ a. Ineffective airway clearance

_____ b. Constipation

_____ c. Impaired gas exchange

_____ d. Acute and chronic pain

_____ e. Noncompliance

_____ f. Nausea

_____ g. Anxiety

_____ h. Fear

_____ i. Impaired oral mucous membranes

5. Write one expected outcome for each of the nursing diagnoses you chose in question 4.

Exercise 3

 CD-ROM Activity—Data Collection

 30 minutes

- Sign in to work at Pacific View Regional Hospital on the Medical-Surgical Floor for Period of Care 3. (*Note:* If you are already in the virtual hospital from a previous exercise, click on **Leave the Floor** and then **Restart the Program** to get to the sign-in window.)
- From the Patient List, select Patricia Newman (Room 406).
- Click on **Get Report** and read the note.
- Click on **Go to Nurses' Station**.
- Click on **Chart** and then on **406**.
- Click on the tab for the **Nursing Admission** and read the admission pages.

The more data you have about your patients, the better care you can deliver. You should know not only about a patient's physical condition but also about his or her living situation, financial stresses, support system, and specific psychosocial problems or concerns. It is important to check what medications the patient was taking at home, just in case a medication for a chronic disorder should be continued in the hospital. You may discover that since a different physician from the patient's primary doctor is caring for the patient, a medication that is necessary has been overlooked. Compare what medications the patient was taking at home with those listed on the MAR or in the orders.

1. What medications was Patricia Newman taking at home?

2. Patricia Newman says her religion is _____ and she _____ like to see the chaplain.

3. She states that she smokes _____.

4. Does it appear that Patricia Newman practices "preventive health care" by obtaining immunizations, doing breast self-exams, and living a healthy lifestyle?

5. What does Patricia Newman indicate is her goal of this hospitalization?

6. Patricia Newman says her normal bowel pattern is _____.

7. What sleep aid does she say she uses?

8. Does she have any hearing or vision difficulties or impairments?

9. Describe Patricia Newman's family relationships.

Exercise 4

CD-ROM Activity—Assessment

15 minutes

- Sign in to work at Pacific View Regional Hospital on the Medical-Surgical Floor for Period of Care 3. (*Note:* If you are already in the virtual hospital from a previous exercise, click on **Leave the Floor** and then **Restart the Program** to get to the sign-in window.)
- From the Patient List, select Patricia Newman (Room 406).
- Click on **Go to Nurses' Station**.
- Click on Room **406**.
- Click on **Take Vital Signs**.

1. Patricia Newman's current vital sign measurements are:

BP _____ SpO$_2$ _____ T _____ HR _____ RR _____ Pain level _____

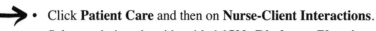 • Click **Patient Care** and then on **Nurse-Client Interactions**.

• Select and view the video titled **1500: Discharge Planning**. (*Note*: Check the virtual clock to see whether enough time has elapsed. You can use the fast forward feature to advance the time by two-minute intervals if the video is not yet available. Then click on **Patient Care** and **Nurse-Client Interactions** to refresh the screen.)

2. What concerns and problems did you discover from the interaction?

Read in Chapter 22 of your textbook about assessment of the chest, heart, and lungs.

• Since Patricia Newman's main problems are respiratory, click on **Physical Assessment** and then on **Chest**. Choose each subcategory of the chest assessment (the green boxes) in turn and record your findings below.

3.

Chest Assessment
   Integumentary

   Cardiovascular

   Breasts

   Respiratory

   Musculoskeletal

4. Considering the data you have gathered for Patricia Newman, identify the four NANDA nursing diagnoses that are priorities for her.

Diagnostic Testing

∞ **Reading Assignment:** Diagnostic Tests and Specimen Collection (Chapter 24)

Patients: Harry George, Medical-Surgical Floor, Room 401
Piya Jordan, Medical-Surgical Floor, Room 403

Objectives:

- Recognize abnormal laboratory values.
- Provide pre- and posttest teaching.
- Recall the proper patient preparation for various diagnostic tests.
- Explain the purpose of various diagnostic tests.
- Explain what to expect during various diagnostic tests.

Diagnostic testing is a cornerstone of medical care. Although the physician orders the tests to be done, it is the nurse who prepares the patient, carries out needed pretest procedures, cares for the patient after the test, and does most of the teaching regarding the purpose of the test and what to expect.

You must learn what factors can interfere with the accuracy of a laboratory test so that money is not spent on a test when the result will not be reliable. Patients are often needlessly fearful of a test because they don't understand how it is done or why it is being done. The nurse must teach the patient about the test and answer any questions.

If a patient is to be away from the unit for several diagnostic tests, you must plan how you will accomplish the necessary care for the patient during the time the patient is on the floor. If you call, many diagnostic centers will tell you what time the patient will be leaving the unit for a particular procedure or test.

Remember: Most times, physicians prefer to give test results to patients themselves. Be sure you know the physician's preference on this matter.

Exercise 1

 CD-ROM Activity—Exploring Laboratory Values

 30 minutes

- Sign in to work at Pacific View Regional Hospital on the Medical-Surgical Floor for Period of Care 3. (*Note:* If you are already in the virtual hospital from a previous exercise, click on Leave the Floor and then Restart the Program to get to the sign-in window.)
- From the Patient List, select Harry George (Room 401).
- Click on **Go to Nurses' Station** and then on **Chart**.
- Click on **401** for Harry George's chart; then select the **Physician's Orders** tab.

1. Identify the laboratory and diagnostic tests ordered for Harry George during this hospitalization. Mark your choices with an X.

_____ a. Blood culture

_____ b. Ventilation perfusion scan

_____ c. CBC

_____ d. Chem 20

_____ e. Pulmonary function tests

_____ f. Bone scan

_____ g. Arterial blood gas

_____ h. Amylase and lipase

_____ i. Culture and sensitivity of wound

_____ j. KUB

_____ k. Clotting studies

_____ l. Folic acid level

_____ m. Alcohol level

_____ n. Chest x-ray

2. When a blood chemistry panel is ordered, there is a requirement that _____

be withheld for _____ hours. (*Hint:* See page 392 in your textbook.)

→ • Click on the **Laboratory Reports** tab and scroll to the urinalysis results.

3. Below, list the values for Harry George's urinalysis. Consider how these findings compare with the normals. Underline any value that is not normal.

Color

Character

Specific gravity

Acetone, ketones

Glucose

Protein

Nitrite

Occult blood

pH

Micro cells:
  Erythrocytes

  Leukocytes

  Bacteria

4. A wound culture was ordered for Harry George. Which of the following must the nurse do when obtaining a wound culture? (*Hint:* See Skill 24-5 on pages 413-414 in your textbook.)
   a. Cleanse the entire wound thoroughly.
   b. Insert the sterile swab into the area where drainage is occurring.
   c. Put on exam gloves before opening swab container.
   d. Swab at least two sites in the wound with one swab.

5. Harry George has a bone scan (radionuclide study) ordered for the left foot. Which of the following statements by the nurse are appropriate in the teaching process to prepare him for the scan? Select all that apply. (*Hint:* See page 404 in your textbook.)

   _____ a. "You must be NPO for 8 hours prior to the scan."

   _____ b. "A radioactive substance is injected into a vein."

   _____ c. "You will be isolated while the radioactive substance is in your body."

   _____ d. "There will be a delay before the scan while the radionuclide is absorbed by the bone."

   _____ e. "You will be asked to empty your bladder after the scan."

   _____ f. "You will be radioactive for 24 hours."

   _____ g. "You will not be radioactive or a danger to others in the vicinity."

➜ • Still in the **Laboratory Reports** section of Harry George's chart, scroll back to find his Hematology results.

6. A complete blood count is often performed either to determine the presence of an infection in the body or to track whether treatment is clearing up an infection. When evaluating the CBC for signs of infection, you would check the number of

_____ and the number of _____. Are the

values abnormal in Harry George's CBCs? _____ (*Hint:* See page 391 and Table 24-2 on page 392 in your textbook.)

➜ • Scroll to the Chemistry section of the Laboratory Reports.

7. What was Harry George's glucose level? _____ The normal range for blood glucose

is _____. Harry George is diabetic. (*Hint:* See Table 24-3 on page 398 in your textbook.)

➜ • Scroll through the Chemistry section of the laboratory reports to find the albumin results.

8. Albumin is one measure of nutritional status of the body. Harry George's albumin level was

_____. The normal range for albumin is _____. Harry George is at risk for poor wound healing because of his albumin level. (*Hint:* See page 398 in your textbook.)

➜ • Click on **Return to Nurses' Station** and then on **MAR**. Choose tab **401** for Harry George's MAR.

9. The first medication listed on Harry George's MAR is _____. This is an antibiotic, and it has a narrow therapeutic range. Peak and trough levels are ordered to track the amount of drug in Harry George's bloodstream.

➜ • Click on **Return to Nurses' Station**; then click on the **Drug** icon in the lower left corner.
 • Use the scroll button to find gentamicin in the drug listings. Read the information and note the therapeutic range for the peak and trough drug levels.
 • Click on **Return to Nurses' Station** and then on **Chart**. Open chart **401** and click again on **Laboratory Reports**. Scroll down to the Drug Monitoring section of the reports.

10. Harry George's peak gentamicin level is _____. The trough level is

_____. Normal therapeutic peak range for gentamicin is

_____, and normal therapeutic trough range is _____.

Toxicity occurs at a peak level greater than _____. If the drug is given at toxic levels over a period of time, there is risk for nephrotoxicity, ototoxicity, and neurotoxicity. When the lab values are in the toxic range, the physician would be notified and the next dose of the drug would be withheld or adjusted or another antibiotic would be substituted.

Exercise 2

 CD-ROM Activity—Diagnostic Tests and Other Laboratory Tests

 45 minutes

- Sign in to work at Pacific View Regional Hospital on the Medical-Surgical Floor for Period of Care 3. (*Note:* If you are already in the virtual hospital from a previous exercise, click on **Leave the Floor** and then **Restart the Program** to get to the sign-in window.)
- From the Patient List, select Piya Jordan (Room 403).
- Click on **Go to Nurses' Station** and then on **403**.
- Read the Initial Observation.
- Click on **Chart** and then on **403**; click on the **Physician's Orders** tab.
- Read the orders, noting the laboratory and diagnostic tests that were ordered for Piya Jordan.

Piya Jordan was admitted with abdominal pain, and her diagnostic workup included several tests.

 1. Match each test name with the appropriate type of test. (*Hint:* Review Chapter 24, especially Tables 24-3 and 24-4, in your textbook.)

Test Name	Type of Test
_____ CT abdomen	a. Blood chemistry
_____ Urinalysis	b. Blood hematology
_____ Hemoglobin and hematocrit	c. Urine test
_____ KUB and upright	d. Computer enhanced x-ray
_____ Chem 7	e. X-ray
_____ PT/INR	f. Blood clotting study
_____ Chest PA and Lat	g. Blood drug monitoring
_____ Digoxin level	h. Blood serology test
_____ Liver function	
_____ Blood type and crossmatch (T & C)	

2. What does a computed tomography scan show? (*Hint:* See Table 24-1 in your textbook.)

3. A KUB is an _____ that shows the

_____. (*Hint:* See page 404 in your textbook.)

→ • Click on the **Diagnostic Tests** tab of the chart and read through the reports.

4. On the report of the CT of the abdomen, what was the impression of the radiologist?

5. The chest x-ray report for Piya Jordan was:
   a. normal.
   b. abnormal.

→ • Click on the **Laboratory Reports** tab in Piya Jordan's chart.

6. The current value for hemoglobin is _____.

   The current value for hematocrit is _____.

   The normal range for hemoglobin is _____.

   The normal range for hematocrit is _____.

   Piya Jordan is _____.

→ • Click on **Return to Room 403** and then on **MAR**. Select tab **403**. Note the digoxin order.
 • Click on **Return to Room 403** and then on the **Drug** icon in the lower left corner. Scroll to digoxin and read about this drug. Note the therapeutic range.

7. Piya Jordan has atrial fibrillation, which is being treated with digoxin. Digoxin has a narrow

   therapeutic range. Piya Jordan has digoxin _____ ordered to be given daily.

   Piya Jordan's digoxin level is _____. The therapeutic range for digoxin is

   _____. Piya Jordan has a _____ level of digoxin
   in her body. Signs to watch for with digoxin toxicity are anorexia, nausea, headache, confusion, yellow- or green-colored vision, and seeing halos around lights.

→ • Once again, click on **Return to Room 403** and then on **Chart**.
 • Choose chart **403** and click on **Laboratory Reports**.
 • Scroll to the Chemistry section and find the potassium level. Low potassium may contribute
   to digoxin toxicity.

8. Piya Jordan's potassium level is _____. The normal range for potassium is

   _____. Piya Jordan is _____
   on potassium. (*Hint:* See Appendix 4 on page 842 in your textbook.) You must memorize
   the normal values for this electrolyte.)

→ • Click on **Return to Room 403** and then on **MAR**. Select tab **403**.

9. How much potassium is Piya Jordan receiving?

→ • One final time, click on **Return to Room 403**.
   • Click on **Chart** and then on **403**.
   • Select the **Laboratory Reports** tab and scroll down to the Special Tests section.

10. Piya Jordan's blood type is _____.

11

Nutrition, Fluid, and Electrolytes

Reading Assignment: Fluid, Electrolyte, and Acid-Base Balance (Chapter 25)
Concepts of Basic Nutrition and Cultural Considerations
(Chapter 26)
Diet Therapy and Assisted Feeding (Chapter 27)

Patients: Piya Jordan, Medical-Surgical Floor, Room 403
Pablo Rodriguez, Medical-Surgical Floor, Room 405

Objectives:

- Identify nutritional components needed for healing.
- Choose appropriate foods for basic therapeutic diets.
- Perform teaching for various therapeutic/restricted diets.
- Recognize abnormal electrolyte values.
- Recognize risks of selected electrolyte imbalances.

Fluid balance is extremely important. The body needs water in order for the chemical and enzyme reactions to take place that keep the body functioning correctly. When water is out of balance, electrolytes are usually out of balance also. If electrolytes get too far out of balance, the patient can die. Acid-base balance abnormalities affect the way the body and its organs function. Every attempt is made to keep the body within a normal acid-base range. It is important for nurses to recognize signs that the blood is too alkaline or too acid. The very young and the elderly are especially prone to fluid and electrolyte imbalances.

Although most hospitals have a dietitian who works with patients on special needs, it is the nurse who performs the majority of the dietary teaching and reinforces the dietitian's instructions. Often it is the nurse who does in-depth teaching so that the patient understands why the diet is necessary and what it is supposed to do.

Patients who have undergone surgery, experienced trauma, or have a serious illness need extra nutrients to promote healing. The nurse should encourage intake when the patient's appetite lags. Often when a patient won't eat, it is because the diet is not what the patient normally eats at home. A patient's cultural food preferences should be accommodated as much as possible. If the dietary department cannot accommodate the patient, having family or friends bring food may be necessary. Of course, you must make certain that foods brought in are not contraindicated for the patient. It is always a good idea to make certain that the patient is not NPO for a test before telling family members that it is okay to give outside food to the patient.

Exercise 1

 CD-ROM Activity—Individual Nutritional Needs

 30 minutes

- Sign in to work at Pacific View Regional Hospital on the Medical-Surgical Floor for Period of Care 3. (*Note:* If you are already in the virtual hospital from a previous exercise, click on **Leave the Floor** and then **Restart the Program** to get to the sign-in window.)
- From the Patient List, select Piya Jordan (Room 403).
- Click on **Go to Nurses' Station**.
- Click on **Chart** and then on **403**.

1. In the last lesson you determined that Piya Jordan is anemic. She is NPO at present, but when eating again, she will need dietary counseling. She has just had major surgery and healing should be promoted. When healing from surgery or a major wound, the body needs

   more _____. (*Hint:* See page 445 in your textbook.) The average DRI for this

   diet component for the healthy adult is _____.

2. Considering that Piya Jordan is Asian-American and may favor Asian foods, what would be a plant source of protein for her?

3. Which vitamin plays a vital role in healing and should be increased in Piya Jordan's diet once she is eating? (*Hint:* See Table 26-6 in your textbook.)

4. Which of the following data are essential when assessing nutritional status? Mark your choices with an X. (*Hint:* See pages 459-461 in your textbook.)

   _____ a. Age

   _____ b. Hours of sleep per night

   _____ c. Height

   _____ d. Occupation

   _____ e. Income level

_____ f. Number of family members

_____ g. Usual diet

_____ h. Activity

_____ i. Food preferences

_____ j. General appearance

_____ k. Weight gain or loss

_____ l. Weight

_____ m. Religion

→ • Click on the **Nursing Admission** tab of the chart and find Piya Jordan's height and weight.

5. Piya Jordan's weight is _____, and her height is _____. Her weight

in pounds is _____.

6. Considering her height and weight, is Piya Jordan's BMI within the acceptable range? What is her BMI? (_Hint:_ See the formula to calculate BMI on page 459 in your textbook.)

→ • Click on **Return to Nurses' Station** and then on **Kardex**.
• Select tab **403** and scroll to the Diet section of the Kardex.

7. What is Piya Jordan's current diet order? What nutrition is she receiving?

8. You've identified a vitamin that Piya Jordan needs to increase in her diet to aid in healing. She will also need additional iron to combat her anemia. Match the following food with the nutrient(s) they will supply. (*Hint:* See Tables 26-6 and 26-8 in your textbook.)

Food	Nutrient(s) Supplied
_____ Orange juice	a. Vitamin C
_____ Red meat	b. Iron
_____ Strawberries	c. Vitamin C and iron
_____ Legumes	
_____ Tomatoes	
_____ Green peppers	
_____ Potatoes	
_____ Whole grains	
_____ Green leafy vegetables	
_____ Fortified cereals	
_____ Grapefruit	

9. Piya Jordan will also need to have sufficient potassium in her diet. Match the following foods with the nutrient(s) they supply. The more foods that supply two or more of the nutrients she requires, the better.

Food	Nutrient(s) Supplied
_____ Bananas	a. Potassium
_____ Oranges	b. Potassium and vitamin C
_____ Broccoli	c. Potassium, vitamin C, and iron
_____ Carrots	d. Potassium and iron
_____ Potatoes	
_____ Meat	
_____ Legumes	
_____ Coffee	

10. After surgery most patients begin eating with a _____ diet and then progress until they are eating normally again.

Exercise 2

  CD-ROM Activity—Fluid and Electrolyte Imbalance

 30 minutes

- Sign in to work at Pacific View Regional Hospital on the Medical-Surgical Floor for Period of Care 3. (*Note:* If you are already in the virtual hospital from a previous exercise, click on **Leave the Floor** and then **Restart the Program** to get to the sign-in window.)
- From the Patient List, select Pablo Rodriguez (Room 405).
- Click on **Get Report** and read the note.

1. What two factors mentioned in report are likely to interfere with Pablo Rodriguez's nutritional intake? (*Hint:* See page 454 in your textbook.)

- Click on **Go to Nurses' Station** and then on **Chart**.
- Select chart **405** and click on the **Emergency Department** tab. Read the entire section.

2. What two fluid and electrolyte problems did Pablo Rodriguez have when admitted to the Emergency Department?

3. Which of the following are signs of dehydration? Mark your choices with an X. (*Hint:* See Table 24-4 on page 424 in your textbook.)

_____ a. Elevated temperature

_____ b. Elevated blood pressure

_____ c. Decreased urine output

_____ d. Increased pulse rate

_____ e. Vomiting

_____ f. Postural hypotension

_____ g. Thick saliva

_____ h. Poor skin turgor

4. What signs of dehydration does Pablo Rodriguez exhibit in the Emergency Department?

→ • Click on the **Laboratory Reports** tab. Scroll down to the Chemistry section and find the electrolyte values.

5. Record Pablo Rodriguez's electrolyte values for the days specified in the table below. Indicate whether each value is normal or abnormal.

	Tues	**Normal/Abnormal**	**Wed**	**Normal/Abnormal**
Sodium				
Potassium				
Calcium				
Phosphate				
Magnesium				

Read in your medical-surgical textbook about carcinoma of the lung. Note where this type of tumor is likely to metastasize.

→ • Click on the **History and Physical** tab of the chart and read through the pages.

6. What risk factor does Pablo Rodriguez have for hypercalcemia?

7. What two signs and symptoms of hypercalcemia does Pablo Rodriguez display?

8. If Pablo Rodriguez's calcium level continues to rise, he will be at risk for life-threatening

———————————.

9. How is Pablo Rodriguez's fluid imbalance treated in the Emergency Department?

It is important to treat Pablo Rodriguez's nausea and vomiting so that he can take in adequate nutrition and stabilize his fluid and electrolytes.

➜ • Click on the **Physician's Orders** tab and note the first medication ordered. Scroll down and note the drug ordered for nausea on Tuesday. Now read all of the physician's orders.

• Click on **Return to Nurses' Station** and then click on the **Drug** icon in the lower left corner. Read about these two drugs that work differently.

10. The drug ordered for Pablo Rodriguez on Wednesday is _____.

On Tuesday, the drug ordered for nausea was _____.

11. Why do you think Neutra-Phos was ordered for Pablo Rodriguez?

12. The diet the physician ordered for Pablo Rodriguez was _____.

 13. Which of the following foods would be allowed on this diet? Mark your choices with an X. (*Hint:* See Chapter 27 and Appendix 5 in your textbook.)

_____ a. Whole milk

_____ b. Lean meat

_____ c. Cheese enchiladas

_____ d. Fish

_____ e. Ice cream

_____ f. Butter

_____ g. Margarine

_____ h. Chili beans

_____ i. Plain vegetables

Exercise 3

 CD-ROM Activity—Calculating and Evaluating Intake and Output

15 minutes

When patients are dehydrated, it is important to monitor their intake and output.

- Sign in to work at Pacific View Regional Hospital on the Medical-Surgical Floor for Period of Care 3. (*Note:* If you are already in the virtual hospital from a previous exercise, click on **Leave the Floor** and then **Restart the Program** to get to the sign-in window.)
- From the Patient List, select Pablo Rodriguez (Room 405).
- Click on **Go to Nurses' Station**.
- Click on **EPR** and then on **Login**.
- Choose **405** in the Patient box and select **Intake and Output** in the Category box.
- Scroll back to the Wednesday 0700 I&O results.

1. The shift intake for Pablo Rodriguez is _____.

   His output was _____.

2. Do you think that this indicates he is rehydrating? Explain.

- Using the scroll buttons, note the I&O amounts from 0700 to the current time.

3. Record the patient's I&O amounts below.

   Intake: _____ Output: _____ (*Hint:* See Skill 25-1 on page 436 in your textbook.)

4. Is there still a positive intake balance, indicating rehydration?

5. How many hours ago did Pablo Rodriguez last experience vomiting (emesis)?

6. In dehydration, water is drawn out of the cells by _____. (*Hint:* See page 424 in your textbook.)

7. Which of the following items could you offer Pablo Rodriguez to help rehydrate him? Consider his ordered diet and his postnausea status. Mark your choices with an X.

_____ a. Popsicle

_____ b. Soft-boiled egg

_____ c. Nonfat milk

_____ d. Juice (clear)

_____ e. Boullion

_____ f. Milkshake

_____ g. Soft drink

_____ h. Gelatin

_____ i. Sherbet

Once Pablo Rodriguez's nausea is well controlled, you would want to encourage a high-calorie, high-protein diet. Cancer increases the metabolic rate of the body and more calories are needed to prevent weight loss. Protein is needed to promote healing from the side effects of chemotherapy or radiation.

Respiration and Oxygen Delivery

∽ **Reading Assignment:** Fluid, Electrolyte, and Acid-Base Balance (Chapter 25)
Assisting with Respiration and Oxygen Delivery (Chapter 28)

Patients: Jacquline Catanazaro, Medical-Surgical Floor, Room 402
Patricia Newman, Medical-Surgical Floor, Room 406

Objectives:

- Recognize abnormalities in SpO_2 and other vital signs that indicate a respiratory problem.
- Analyze trends in respiratory data.
- Identify signs of hypoxia.
- Safely administer oxygen.
- State the purpose of various respiratory drugs.
- Assist the patient with respiratory treatments.

The supply of oxygen to the body's cells is dependent on the proper function of the respiratory and cardiovascular systems. The respiratory system, through ventilation and diffusion, exchanges gases between the blood interface in the lungs and the external air. The cardiovascular system provides perfusion of the oxygen to the cells. Expanded alveoli and clear bronchioles that are unimpeded by secretions are necessary for proper gas exchange to take place. Various disorders can affect either the lungs' capability to exchange gases or the vascular system's ability to carry gases to and from the cells of the body. Additionally, the patient's lifestyle, environmental factors, and medications contribute to his or her respiratory or cardiac status.

When respiratory problems occur, there are specific signs and symptoms that indicate a problem. It is crucial to the patient's well-being that the nurse be able to evaluate changes in a patient's respiratory or cardiac status. Critical thinking and consequent quick intervention, often with relatively simple measures, can avert a serious problem.

Exercise 1

 CD-ROM Activity—Respiratory Assessment

 30 minutes

- Sign in to work at Pacific View Regional Hospital on the Medical-Surgical Floor for Period of Care 1. (*Note:* If you are already in the virtual hospital from a previous exercise, click on **Leave the Floor** and then **Restart the Program** to get to the sign-in window.)
- From the Patient List, select Jacquline Catanazaro (Room 402).
- Click on **Get Report** for Jacquline Catanazaro and read the note.
- Click on **Go to Nurses' Station** and then on **402** to go to the patient's room.
- Read the **Initial Observations** and **Clinical Alerts**.
- Click on **Patient Care** and proceed with a brief, focused respiratory assessment. First, click on **Chest** and then select **Respiratory** and **Musculoskeletal** in turn from the specific subcategories (green boxes).

1.

Focused Assessment—Chest

Respiratory

Musculoskeletal

Go online and log in to the Evolve website (http://evolve.elsevier.com/deWit/). From the left-hand menu, select the **Course Material** folder and click on **Audio Clips**. Listen to breath sounds that are similar to the ones Jacquline Catanazaro is exhibiting. (*Hint:* Check that the speakers are on and that the volume is turned up sufficiently. If you don't have Internet access, the same audio clips can be found on the Student CD that was bound into your *Fundamental Concepts and Skills for Nursing* textbook, 2nd edition.)

 2. Is Jacquline Catanazaro's SpO$_2$ within normal limits? (*Hint:* See Skill 28-1 on page 495 in your textbook.)

3. Review Table 22-4 on page 365 of your textbook. How would you describe the sound of wheezing?

 • Click on **Chart** and then on **402**.
   • Click on the **History and Physical** tab. Read through the physician's History and Physical.

   4. What do you find in the History and Physical that could account for the cause of this wheezing?

Read in your medical-surgical textbook about asthma, its signs and symptoms, triggering factors, and treatment.

• Click on **Return to Room 402**.
   • Click on **Take Vital Signs** and note the respiratory rate.

   5. Jacquline Catanazaro's respiratory rate is _____. The normal adult respiratory rate is

   _____.

• Click on **Patient Care** and then on **Nurse-Client Interactions**.
   • Select and view the video titled **0730: Intervention—Airway**. (*Note*: Check the virtual clock to see whether enough time has elapsed. You can use the fast forward feature to advance the time by two-minute intervals if the video is not yet available. Then click on **Patient Care** and **Nurse-Client Interactions** to refresh the screen.)

   6. What does Jacquline Catanazaro tell the nurse?

   7. What does the nurse tell Jacquline Catanazaro is the current plan?

• Click on **Chart** and then on **402**. Select the **Laboratory Reports** tab. Scroll down to the Arterial Blood Gas section.

8. In the table below, record Jacquline Catanazaro's arterial blood gas results for the times specified.

ABGs	Mon 1030	Wed 0730
PaO$_2$		
O$_2$ sat		
PaCO$_2$		
pH		

9. Based on the blood gas values above, what is Jacquline Catanazaro's acid-base abnormality? (*Hint:* See Table 25-6 on page 430 in your textbook.)

Exercise 2

 CD-ROM Activity—Respiratory Treatments

 15 minutes

- Sign in to work at Pacific View Regional Hospital on the Medical-Surgical Floor for Period of Care 1. (*Note:* If you are already in the virtual hospital from a previous exercise, click on **Leave the Floor** and then **Restart the Program** to get to the sign-in window.)
- From the Patient List, select Jacquline Catanazaro (Room 402).
- Click on **Get Report** for Jacquline Catanazaro and read the note.
- Click on **Go to Nurses' Station** and then on **Chart**.
- Select the chart for **402**. Click on the **Physician's Orders** tab and read the most current orders.

 1. What is the purpose of the nebulizer treatment that is ordered for Jacquline Catanazaro? (*Hint:* See pages 520-523 in your textbook.) What medication is ordered?

→ • Click on **Return to Nurses' Station** and then click on the **Drug** icon in the lower left corner. Scroll to the drug ordered for the nebulizer treatment and read about it.

2. The normal adult dosage for a nebulizer treatment of this medication is _____.

3. This drug has many side effects. Which problems that Jacquline Catanazaro is already displaying might be exacerbated by this drug?

_____ a. Stuffy head

_____ b. Chest tightness

_____ c. Nervousness

_____ d. Headache

_____ e. Tachypnea

_____ f. Restlessness

→ • Click on **Return to Nurses' Station** and then on **MAR**. Select tab **402** and find the three drugs Jacquline Catanazaro is to receive by inhaler (puffs or MDI). Record these drugs in the table in question 4.

• Once again, click on **Return to Nurses' Station** and then on the **Drug** icon. Find each of the three drugs you listed in the table below. As you read about each drug, record its purpose in the table.

4. In the table below, identify the three drugs Jacquline Catanazaro is to receive by inhaler. List the purpose of each of these drugs as well.

Inhaler Medication	Purpose

→ • You should have noticed in the MAR that Jacquline Catanazaro is also receiving prednisone. Read about this drug in the Drug Guide.

5. How do you think that prednisone helps a person with asthma?

Exercise 3

 CD-ROM Activity—Oxygen Therapy

 30 minutes

• Sign in to work at Pacific View Regional Hospital on the Medical-Surgical Floor for Period of Care 1. (*Note:* If you are already in the virtual hospital from a previous exercise, click on **Leave the Floor** and then **Restart the Program** to get to the sign-in window.)
• From the Patient List, select Patricia Newman (Room 406).
• Click on **Get Report** for Patricia Newman and read the note.
• Click on **Go to Nurses' Station** and then on **Chart.**
• Click on the chart for **406** and then on the **Physician's Orders** tab. Read the orders.

1. The physician has ordered oxygen at _____ by nasal cannula for Patricia

   Newman. The normal range for oxygen flow is _____.

2. An oxygen flow rate of 2 liters/min by nasal cannula provides the patient with

   _____% oxygen.

 3. Although Patricia Newman's oxygen saturation is only 88%, the nurse does not increase the flow. Why is it unwise to increase the flow for this patient? (*Hint:* See the History and Physical to read about any long-standing disorders she has. Also see page 506 in your textbook.)

4. Which of the following nursing actions are appropriate when a patient has oxygen ordered by nasal cannula? Mark your choices with an X.

_____ a. Check nares to see that they are unobstructed.

_____ b. Observe for excoriation on the nose.

_____ c. Humidification is required if the flow rate is greater than 2 liters/min.

_____ d. Humidification is always required when an O_2 cannula is used.

_____ e. Cleanse the nares each shift and check for signs of irritation.

_____ f. The cannula may be removed to make eating meals easier.

_____ g. Check the oxygen flow rate each time the room is entered to be certain it is set properly.

_____ h. Check the back of the ears and lobes for signs of irritation each shift.

5. When a patient has oxygen ordered, safety measures must be instituted. What two things must the nurse do when instituting oxygen therapy?

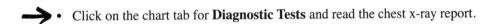 • Click on the chart tab for **Diagnostic Tests** and read the chest x-ray report.

6. What does the impression note on the chest x-ray report say?

 7. All patients with a respiratory ailment must be watched for signs of hypoxia. Which of the following is frequently the earliest sign of hypoxia? (*Hint:* See page 494 in your textbook.)
   a. Constant cough
   b. Stridor
   c. Substernal retractions
   d. Restlessness

8. Hypoxia and respiratory insufficiency cause different signs and symptoms, depending on how long the patient has been hypoxic. Match each stage of hypoxia with the signs or symptoms common during that period. (*Hint:* See Table 28-2 on page 494 of your textbook.)

Sign or Symptom	**Stage of Hypoxia**
_____ Cyanosis	a. Early
_____ Anxiety	b. Late
_____ Tachypnea	c. Latest
_____ Drop in blood pressure	
_____ Confusion	
_____ Muscle retractions	
_____ Stridor	
_____ Sitting up to breathe	
_____ Dysrhythmia	

9. In a person with emphysema, ineffective coughing spasms may lead to _____

of the alveoli and may precipitate _____ of the airways. (*Hint:* See page 501 in your textbook.)

10. Patricia Newman has pneumonia and a productive cough. She must cough effectively in order to clear her lungs of secretions. What type of coughing would you institute with her? (*Hint:* See page 501 in your textbook.)

11. Describe the instructions you would give Patricia Newman for this type of coughing.

13

Activity, Mobility, and Skin Care

Reading Assignment: Infection Control in the Hospital and Home (Chapter 17)
Lifting, Moving, and Positioning Patients (Chapter 18)
Assisting with Hygiene, Personal Care, Skin Care, and the
Prevention of Pressure Ulcers (Chapter 19)
Promoting Musculoskeletal Function (Chapter 39)

Patients: Clarence Hughes, Medical-Surgical Floor, Room 404
Harry George, Medical-Surgical Floor, Room 401
Patricia Newman, Medical-Surgical Floor, Room 406

Objectives:

- Recognize areas of pressure that occur with different patient positions.
- Recall risk factors that contribute to the formation of pressure ulcers.
- Discuss the effects of immobility on the body's systems.
- Assist patients to use devices that promote mobility.

Exercise of activity is essential to maintaining a healthy body. When extended periods of immobility occur, every system of the body is affected. Regular movement is necessary for joints to maintain their usual range of motion. Illness and injury affect mobility and activity tolerance. When a patient cannot move certain joints, the nurse must help with therapy and exercises that will preserve or improve joint function. Physical therapists work with patients to promote proper joint function, to help maintain muscle strength, and to help with regaining ambulation and independence.

Immobility of even a few days' duration can cause problems in multiple body systems. A major concern when immobility occurs is the risk for respiratory problems. Your textbook tells you that "Activity causes people to breathe more deeply, expanding their lungs and encouraging clearing of normal secretions." Frequent turning, range of motion exercises, and deep breathing and coughing exercises help to prevent respiratory complications.

Activity helps muscles contract and assists circulation as the muscles press on the vein walls, forcing blood back toward the heart. The digestive system does not function as well when the body is immobile. A major problem of immobility is the risk for pressure ulcers. Pressure ulcers can occur within a very short period of time if a patient is positioned for too long without turning. Great attention must be paid to skin care, inspection of pressure points, and preventive measures to avoid pressure ulcers.

Exercise 1

  CD-ROM Activity

30 minutes

- Sign in to work at Pacific View Regional Hospital on the Medical-Surgical Floor for Period of Care 2. (*Note:* If you are already in the virtual hospital from a previous exercise, click on **Leave the Floor** and then **Restart the Program** to get to the sign-in window.)
- From the Patient List, select Clarence Hughes (Room 404).
- Click on **Get Report** and note pertinent information given in the report.
- Click on **Go to Nurses' Station** and then on Room **404**.
- Read the **Initial Observations** and the **Clinical Alerts** notes.
- Click on **Chart** and then on **404**. Select the **Physician's Orders** tab.

1. From an earlier lesson, you know that Clarence Hughes had a left total knee arthroplasty (replacement) on Monday. What are the current activity orders for Clarence Hughes?

 2. Clarence Hughes will be in a supine or semi-Fowler's position during the day in order to use the CPM device; thus he will not be able to turn to his side. However, at night he may turn to the right side. Below, match the pressure areas pertinent to a supine position and those pertinent to a side-lying position. (*Hint:* See page 277 in your textbook.)

Pressure Area	Position
_____ Sacrum/coccyx	a. Supine position
_____ Occiput	b. Side-lying position
_____ Dorsal/thoracic area	
_____ Ischial tuberosity	
_____ Posterior knee	
_____ Malleolus	
_____ Lateral knee	
_____ Ilium	
_____ Trochanter	
_____ Shoulder	
_____ Elbow	
_____ Heel	
_____ Shoulder blade	

3. When an area of redness is observed after turning a patient, what is the appropriate action? Mark your choice with an X. (*Hint:* See page 278 in your textbook.)

_____ a. Massage the area.

_____ b. Reassess the area in 30-45 minutes.

_____ c. Immediately check to see whether the area will blanch.

_____ d. Apply a hot pack to the area.

4. If you turn Clarence Hughes from a side-lying to a supine position during the night and you notice a reddened area on the right hip and the area does not blanch when you go back to

check on it in an hour, you would chart that he has a _____ pressure ulcer. (*Hint:* See page 279 in your textbook.)

5. If a stage 1 pressure ulcer has formed, which of the following should you do? (*Hint:* See p. 763 in your textbook.)
a. Leave the area open to the air.
b. Apply a hydrocolloid dressing.
c. Apply a gauze dressing.
d. Apply a transparent film dressing.

6. What are the purposes of using passive continuous motion after joint replacement? (*Hint:* See page 791 in your textbook.)

7. When Clarence Hughes ambulates, he uses a walker. Which of the following would indicate to you that the walker is the right height for the patient? (*Hint:* See page 805 in your textbook.)
a. The hand rests are at the level of the patient's hips.
b. The patient's elbows are bent at 35-degree angles when the hands are on the hand grips.
c. The front bar is parallel and even with the patient's waist.
d. The patient's elbows are bent at 25-degree angles when the hands are on the hand grips.

8. Clarence Hughes' new knee and its limited range of motion put him at risk for a fall. When he gets up to ambulate, you would teach him to do which of the following? Mark your choices with an X.

_____ a. Sit for a minute or two before standing.

_____ b. Stand still until any dizziness passes before beginning to walk.

_____ c. Wear firm-soled slippers.

_____ d. Lean slightly forward while using the walker.

_____ e. Maintain good, upright posture while ambulating.

_____ f. Ambulate only with someone holding on to him.

9. Because Clarence Hughes has had a knee joint replacement, he is at risk for neurovascular impairment. You should perform a neurovascular assessment on him every shift. Based on

   Clarence Hughes' age, the capillary refill in his toes should be _____.
   (*Hint:* See Table 39-4 on page 793 in your textbook.)

10. Describe how you would check sensation when performing your neurovascular assessment.
    (*Hint:* See page 793 in your textbook.)

11. What are the four effects of immobility on the musculoskeletal system? (*Hint:* See page 785 in your textbook.) Mark your choices with an X.

    _____ a. Renal stones

    _____ b. Venous stasis

    _____ c. Decreased muscle mass and muscle tension

    _____ d. Negative nitrogen balance

    _____ e. Ischemia and necrosis of tissue

    _____ f. Shortening of muscle

    _____ g. Loss of calcium from bone matrix

    _____ h. Decrease in bone weight

    _____ i. Decreased independence

12. Because of the immobility caused by his surgical procedure, Clarence Hughes is at risk for

    the cardiovascular-respiratory complication _____. (*Hint:*
    See Table 39-1 on page 785 of your textbook.) He is at double the risk for this complication because his long bones were involved in the surgery.

13. Clarence Hughes will be transported to the radiology department for a ventilation-perfusion scan. He will be transported by wheelchair. A major safety precaution when transferring a patient into or out of a wheelchair is to:
    a. place the chair to the left of the patient, who is seated on the bed.
    b. place the chair to the right of the patient, who is seated on the bed.
    c. move the leg extensions on the chair to the lowest position.
    d. check to see that the wheel locks are engaged.

Read in your textbook about the complication you identified in question 12.

• Click on **Return to Room 404**.
• Click on **Patient Care** and then on **Chest**.
• Click on each subcategory of the chest assessment in turn (the green boxes).

14. Based on the change-of-shift report, the Initial Observations, the Clinical Alert, and your chest assessment, Clarence Hughes experiences which signs and symptoms of the complication you identified in question 12? Mark your choices with an X.

_____ a. Leaning forward

_____ b. Diaphoresis

_____ c. Coughing

_____ d. Shortness of breath

_____ e. Chest pain

_____ f. Anxiety

_____ g. Tachypnea

_____ h. Production of frothy sputum

Exercise 2

CD-ROM Activity—Pressure Ulcer Risk and Infection

30 minutes

- Sign in to work at Pacific View Regional Hospital on the Medical-Surgical Floor for Period of Care 1. (*Note:* If you are already in the virtual hospital from a previous exercise, click on **Leave the Floor** and then **Restart the Program** to get to the sign-in window.)
- From the Patient List, select Harry George (Room 401).
- Click on **Get Report** and review the note.
- Click on **Go to Nurses' Station** and then on **401**.
- Read the **Initial Observations** and **Clinical Alerts** notes.
- Click on **Chart** and then on **401**. Select the **Physician's Orders** tab.

1. What are the activity and positioning orders for Harry George?

2. When elevating Harry George's foot on pillows, you must be very careful to protect the

_____ from pressure.

- Click on **History and Physical** and read through the form.

3. From the information in the History and Physical, what would you expect Harry George's nutritional status to be?

4. Which of the following factors cause a patient to be at greater risk for a pressure ulcer? (*Hint:* See page 276 in your textbook.) Mark your choices with an X.

_____ a. Continued diaphoresis

_____ b. Obesity

_____ c. Weight loss

_____ d. Incontinence

_____ e. Bed rest

_____ f. Dehydration

_____ g. Confusion

_____ h. Edema

_____ i. Poor nutrition

5. Considering the data you have obtained, how many risk factors does Harry George have for developing a pressure ulcer?

• Click on **Physician's Notes** and determine what organism has caused the infection in Harry George's foot.

6. The organism causing the infection in Harry George's foot is

_____.

• Click on **Return to Room 401** and click on **Patient Care**.
• Perform a focused assessment on Harry George's **Lower Extremities**.

7. Below, record your findings from the focused assessment of Harry George's lower extremities.

Focused Assessment—Lower Extremities

Integumentary

Musculoskeletal

Vascular

Neurologic

→ • Click on **EPR** and then on **Login**.

• Select **401** in the Patient box. Using the drop-down menu next to the Category box, document the assessment you just performed on Harry George.

8. The physician has ordered dressing changes for Harry George's foot. This procedure requires the use of standard precautions. Which of the following protective barrier items will be required to perform this dressing change? Mark your choices with an X.

_____ a. Gloves

_____ b. Gown

_____ c. Mask

_____ d. Goggles

_____ e. Biohazard discard bag

_____ f. Private room

9. There are special criteria for transmission-based precautions in the hospital. Harry George's wound would require _____ precautions. (*Hint:* See Table 17-4, p. 229 in your textbook.)

10. When performing a dressing change for Harry George, you must adhere to principles of aseptic technique. Indicate the actions that adhere to aseptic principles while performing this dressing change. (*Hint:* See Skill 38-1, pages 768-769 in your textbook.) Mark your choices with an X.

_____ a. Do not use dressings that have been opened but left in the room.

_____ b. Set up the sterile field above your waist height.

_____ c. Open sterile pack wrappers away from the body.

_____ d. Open the sterile glove pack on your sterile field.

_____ e. Place the discard bag at the back edge of the sterile field.

_____ f. Once gloved, keep your hands in sight.

Exercise 3

CD-ROM Activity—Physical Therapy to Increase Mobility and Endurance

15 minutes

Recall from the earlier lessons that Patricia Newman suffers from emphysema and was hospitalized for pneumonia. She has not been eating well and is fatigued most of the time. The physician has ordered a physical therapy consult to determine a program to increase her mobility and endurance.

• Sign in to work at Pacific View Regional Hospital on the Medical-Surgical Floor for Period of Care 4. (*Note:* If you are already in the virtual hospital from a previous exercise, click on **Leave the Floor** and then **Restart the Program** to get to the sign-in window.)

• Click on **Chart** and then on **406**. Click on the **Consultations** tab and scroll to the PT/OT Consult. Read through the consultation notes. (*Remember:* You are not able to visit patients or administer medications during Period of Care 4. You are able to review patients' records only.)

1. The plan states that Patricia Newman is to begin her "pulmonary rehabilitation" plan by

walking _____ minutes _____ times a day.

2. Patricia Newman is to walk _____ (independently/with assistance) for her activity plan.

3. What is the goal of the physical therapy program?

4. Is there to be stair climbing included in the plan?

5. What parameters would need to be monitored when Patricia Newman starts the walking plan?

6. For which of the following activities does Patricia Newman require moderate assistance? Mark your choice with an X.

   _____   a. Bathing

   _____   b. Dressing

   _____   c. Toileting

   _____   d. Grooming

   _____   e. Eating

7. What might help her to need less assistance with this daily activity task?

8. The recommendations of the dietitian should be interwoven with the physical therapy plan. Why?

9. How might the exercise plan help prevent further bouts of pneumonia? (*Hint:* Use critical thinking for this question.)

Elimination

✎ **Reading Assignment:** Promoting Urinary Elimination (Chapter 29)
Promoting Bowel Elimination (Chapter 30)

Patients: Piya Jordan, Medical-Surgical Floor, Room 403
Pablo Rodriguez, Medical-Surgical Floor, Room 405
Harry George, Medical-Surgical Floor, Room 401

Objectives:

- Identify factors in patient scenarios that interfere with normal urination.
- Adequately assess elimination status of patients.
- Recognize abnormal laboratory values for urine tests.
- Describe proper urinary catheter care.
- Describe factors that influence bowel elimination for patients.
- List specific factors that contribute to elimination problems in patients.

To function properly, the body must eliminate the waste products of metabolism. Elimination patterns are affected by lifestyle choices and habits; therefore patterns vary from one person to another. Alterations in either bowel or urinary elimination can signal changes in other body systems. Good nursing care always involves assessment of urinary and bowel elimination. Knowledge of normal elimination function, recognition of normal and abnormal variations, and a sensitivity to patient needs is essential to good nursing care. It is important to remember than an alteration in urinary or bowel elimination may cause great embarrassment to the patient.

While a patient is in the hospital, additional factors can affect elimination; these factors may include medications, changes in diet and activity level, surgery, and preparations for diagnostic tests (e.g., fasting, ingesting dye substances). During a patient's hospital stay, assessment of both urinary and bowel elimination should be continual. Attending to a dependent patient's elimination needs in a timely fashion is very important to the patient's well-being and recovery.

Exercise 1

 CD-ROM Activity—Urinary Catheter Care

 30 minutes

- Sign in to work at Pacific View Regional Hospital on the Medical-Surgical Floor for Period of Care 1. (*Note:* If you are already in the virtual hospital from a previous exercise, click on **Leave the Floor** and then **Restart the Program** to get to the sign-in window.)
- From the Patient List, select Piya Jordan (Room 403).
- Click on **Get Report** and review the report notes.
- Click on **Go to Nurses' Station**.

Piya Jordan is recovering from a colectomy. She has a Foley catheter in place and as her nurse, you will be providing appropriate urinary catheter care.

1. Each time you enter Piya Jordan's room you should check her urinary status by doing which of the following? Mark your choices with an X.

_____ a. Check the urine in the bag for cloudiness.

_____ b. Switch the collection bag to the opposite side of the bed.

_____ c. Verify that the patient is not lying on the catheter.

_____ d. Irrigate the catheter.

_____ e. Check the connecting tubing to see that it is hanging straight to the collection bag.

_____ f. Make certain that urine is flowing into the bag.

_____ g. Do not raise the collection bag higher than the level of the bladder.

Because Piya Jordan is spending most of her time in bed, and because she has an indwelling catheter, she is at risk for a urinary tract infection. In order to assess her urinary status postoperatively, you need to know her urinalysis results before surgery.

- Click on **Chart** and then on the chart for **403**. Select the **Laboratory Reports** tab.
- Scroll to the urinalysis results and record them in the table in question 2.

2. Record Piya Jordan's urinalysis results below. Mark any abnormal result with an X. (*Hint:* See Table 24-5, page 401 in your textbook.)

Test	Piya Jordan's Results	Abnormal? (X)
Color		
Clarity		
Glucose		
Bilirubin		
Ketones		
Sp. Gr.		
Blood (occult)		
pH		
Protein		
Nitrite		
Micro: WBC		
RBC		
Bacteria		

It appears that Piya Jordan had a urinary tract infection before surgery. She was also dehydrated from vomiting, which can affect the test results. There was no time to treat the infection before her surgery because she had signs and symptoms of a bowel obstruction. The physician has ordered another urinalysis today.

3. To obtain a urine specimen from a patient with an indwelling catheter, you would clamp the

catheter _____ the aspiration port for at least _____ minutes before obtaining the specimen. (*Hint:* See Steps 29-1 on page 533 in your textbook.)

4. You should use a _____-gauge sterile needle and syringe to obtain the urine specimen from the aspiration port.

5. Aspirate _____ mL of urine for the urine specimen.

6. Place the following steps for obtaining the urine specimen in the correct order by numbering from 1 to 12.

_____ Put on gloves.

_____ Open the sterile container.

_____ Label the sterile container.

_____ Check the order.

_____ Clamp off the catheter.

_____ Empty the syringe into the sterile container.

_____ Aspirate the urine from the catheter.

_____ Swab the aspiration port with alcohol.

_____ Insert the needle into the aspiration port.

_____ Instruct the patient about the procedure.

_____ Close the sterile container.

_____ Remove and dispose of the gloves.

7. Changes can occur in urine if it sits at room temperature for very long. If a urine specimen cannot be taken to the laboratory immediately, it should be _____. It is best to send the labeled specimen, packaged in a biohazard bag, to the laboratory immediately.

8. Piya Jordan is at risk for bladder infection for a variety of reasons. Which of the following apply? Mark your choices with an X.

_____ a. Urinary stasis from bed rest and inactivity

_____ b. Bowel colectomy

_____ c. Dehydration from nausea and vomiting before surgery

_____ d. NPO status with intravenous fluid administration

_____ e. Presence of an indwelling catheter

_____ f. Obesity

_____ g. Decreased bladder tone and possible incomplete emptying due to age

9. What is the single most important nursing measure to prevent infection for the patient who has an indwelling catheter? (*Hint:* Use critical thinking for this question.)

 10. What signs and symptoms would you look for that might tell you your patient is experiencing a bladder infection (cystitis)? (*Hint:* See page 530 in your textbook.)

11. People who are prone to recurrent bladder infections should drink a lot of water (2500-3000 mL a day) and should void at least every _____ hours. (*Hint:* See Nursing Care Plan 29-1 on pages 535-536 in your textbook.)

Exercise 2

 CD-ROM Activity—Assisting with Bowel Elimination

 30 minutes

- Sign in to work at Pacific View Regional Hospital on the Medical-Surgical Floor for Period of Care 1. (*Note:* If you are already in the virtual hospital from a previous exercise, click on **Leave the Floor** and then **Restart the Program** to get to the sign-in window.)
- From the Patient List, select Pablo Rodriguez (Room 405).
- Click on **Get Report** and review the notes.
- Click on **Go to Nurses' Station**.
- Click on Room **405** to visit Pablo Rodriguez.
- Read the Initial Observation.
- Click on **MAR** and verify that the page is for Pablo Rodriguez (tab **405**).

1. What medication is Pablo Rodriguez receiving that can cause constipation?

- Click on **Return to Room 405**.
- Click on **Patient Care** and perform an abdominal assessment on Pablo Rodriguez. Record your findings in the chart on the next page.

2. Record your findings from Pablo Rodriguez's abdominal assessment below.

Assessment—Abdomen

Integumentary

Musculoskeletal

Gastrointestinal

→ • Click on **EPR** and on **Login**. Choose **405** in the Patient box. Using the Category drop-down menu, select **Gastrointestinal**. Enter the above findings in the correct columns using the symbols listed for each line.

3. When did Pablo Rodriguez have his last bowel movement? What were the characteristics of his stool? (*Hint:* See earlier entries in the EPR.)

4. Why do you think Pablo Rodriguez is at risk for constipation and fecal impaction?

5. The physician has ordered a mineral oil enema in case Pablo Rodriguez doesn't have a bowel movement by midmorning. When giving a mineral oil enema, you know that it

should be retained for _____ in order to be effective.

• Click on **Exit EPR** and then on **MAR**. (Again, verify that the MAR page is for Pablo Rodriguez.) Note the medications on the MAR that are used to prevent or treat constipation. Click on the **Drug** icon in the lower left corner and look up any medications with which you are unfamiliar.

6. Below, list the medications from Pablo Rodriguez's MAR that treat or prevent constipation. For each medication, list the action and/or use.

Medication	Action/Use

7. If the physician orders a soap suds enema for Pablo Rodriguez, there are specific steps to be followed.

   a. How would you position Pablo Rodriguez to administer the enema?

   b. During a soap suds enema, how should the container be positioned?

c. What is the rationale for running the solution into the patient's body slowly?

d. What should be the temperature of the solution?

Exercise 3

CD-ROM Activity—Measures to Prevent Constipation

30 minutes

- Sign in to work at Pacific View Regional Hospital on the Medical-Surgical Floor for Period of Care 2. (*Note:* If you are already in the virtual hospital from a previous exercise, click on **Leave the Floor** and then **Restart the Program** to get to the sign-in window.)
- From the Patient List, select Harry George (Room 401).
- Click on **Get Report** and review the report note.
- Click on **Go to Nurses' Station**.
- Click on **Kardex** and then on tab **401**. Check what type of activity is ordered for Harry George.
- Click on **Return to Nurses' Station** and then on **Chart**. Click on **401** and then on the tab for **Nurse's Notes**. Read about Harry George's food intake.
- Click on **Return to Nurses' Station** and then on **MAR**. Select tab **401** and note the medications Harry George is taking that could contribute to constipation. (*Hint:* What pain medication is he receiving?)

1. How has Harry George been eating? What factors in his eating pattern could contribute to constipation?

→ • Once again, click on **Return to Nurses' Station** and then on **Chart**. Select the **Expired MARs** and read through them.

2. It appears that Harry George is receiving the pain medication

_____ about every _____ . He has had _____ doses since admission. (*Hint:* Remember to check today's MAR also.)

→ • Click on the chart tab for **Nursing Admission** and review the Elimination section.

3. Harry George's usual bowel pattern is to have a bowel movement _____.

→ • Click on **Return to Nurses' Station** and click on **EPR**. Select **401** in the Patient box. Use the Category drop-down menu to choose **Gastrointestinal**. Use the arrows to scroll backwards to see when Harry George has had a bowel movement.

4. Harry George's last bowel movement was _____. He

_____ (does/does not) appear to be constipated.

5. Harry George's physician has ordered magnesium hydrochloride in case Harry George becomes constipated. How does this medication work? (*Hint:* Use the Drug Guide on the CD-ROM, your pharmacology book, or a nursing drug handbook.)

6. Often biscodyl suppositories are ordered prn in case the patient becomes constipated. How does this suppository work?

7. When administering a biscodyl suppository, you instruct the patient to try to retain it for at

least _____. (*Hint:* See Step 34-2 on page 656 in your textbook.)

8. Many actions can help prevent elimination problems. For each action listed below, indicate whether the action can help prevent constipation (mark with "a"), urinary tract infection (mark with "b"), or both problems (mark with "c").

Action	**Elimination Problem**
_____ Increase fluids to 2500-3000 mL per day	a. Constipation
_____ Increase fresh fruits and vegetables in the diet	b. Urinary tract infection
_____ Exercise every day	c. Constipation and urinary tract infection
_____ Cleanse the perineum from front to back	
_____ Increase vitamin C intake	
_____ Empty the bladder after intercourse	
_____ Pay attention to the urge to defecate	
_____ Use aid such as hot coffee or hot water with lemon juice	
_____ Avoid citrus fruits and juices	
_____ Wear cotton underwear	

Pain, Comfort, and Sleep

Reading Assignment: Cultural and Spiritual Aspects of Patient Care (Chapter 14)
Pain, Comfort, and Sleep (Chapter 31)
Complementary and Alternative Therapies (Chapter 32)

Patients: Clarence Hughes, Medical-Surgical Floor, Room 404
Pablo Rodriguez, Medical-Surgical Floor, Room 405
Kathryn Doyle, Skilled Nursing Floor, Room 503

Objectives:

- Recall the parameters for assessment of pain.
- Discuss the physiologic responses to pain.
- Identify comfort measures to help relieve pain and promote rest.
- Determine precautions for giving various analgesics.
- Develop awareness of cultural and individual responses to pain.
- Choose interventions to help the patient sleep and rest in the hospital.

Pain is a very personal experience. It is difficult to assess a patient's pain objectively. Only the patient can tell you just where his or her pain is located in the body, what it feels like, and how it is affecting functioning. Good pain assessment requires attentive listening, questioning, and close attention to body language. Remember: Pain is what the patient says it is. Each patient's pain is different. You must be careful not to color your perception of what the patient says about pain with your own experiences and cultural beliefs.

Pain has been greatly undertreated in the past and is now a major focus of care for any patient. Nurses must be adept at pain assessment, knowledgeable about pain medication, familiar with the various methods of pain control, and able to implement complementary approaches to pharmacologic treatment of pain. Implementing other comfort measures can be a powerful adjunct to the relief of pain.

Exercise 1

  CD-ROM Activity—Pain Assessment

30 minutes

- Sign in to work at Pacific View Regional Hospital on the Medical-Surgical Floor for Period of Care 1. (*Note:* If you are already in the virtual hospital from a previous exercise, click on **Leave the Floor** and then **Restart the Program** to get to the sign-in window.)
- From the Patient List, select Clarence Hughes (Room 404).
- Click on **Get Report** and read the note.
- Click on **Go to Nurses' Station**.
- Click on Room **404**.
- Read the **Initial Observations** and **Clinical Alerts**.
- Click on **Take Vital Signs** and record them below.

1. Clarence Hughes' current vital sign measurements are:

BP _____ SpO$_2$ _____ T _____ HR _____ RR _____ Pain level _____

- Click on **EPR** and **Login**. Choose **404** in the Patient box. Document the vital signs.

2. Are there any appreciable differences between Clarence Hughes' current vital signs and the previous vital signs?

3. Why is it important to measure the vital signs as part of the pain assessment?

4. According to Table 31-1 on page 587 of your textbook, what four pain factors should be assessed?

   a.

   b.

   c.

   d.

5. What type of pain do you think Clarence Hughes is experiencing? (*Hint:* See pages 585-587 in your textbook.)

→ • Click on **Exit EPR** and then on **MAR**. Verify that the MAR page is for Clarence Hughes.
  • Scroll through the MAR, noting the medications; locate what medication is ordered for pain.

6. The medication ordered for Clarence Hughes' pain is _____.

→ • Click on **Return to Room 404.**
  • Click on **Chart** and then **404**.
  • Select the chart tab for **Expired MARs**.

7. How frequently does the expired MAR indicate that Clarence Hughes has been receiving the pain pills?

8. Clarence Hughes is at risk for what problem(s) while taking this medication?

→ • Click on **Return to Room 404** and then on **EPR**. Click on **Login** and choose **404** in the Patient box. Use the Category drop-down menu to select **Gastrointestinal**.

9. Clarence Hughes had his last bowel movement _____.

10. The notes you have read indicate that his knee and lower leg are swollen. How does this affect the pain level? (*Hint:* Use critical thinking for this question.)

11. When Clarence Hughes' leg is not in the CPM machine, which of the following adjunctive measures might be used to decrease his pain? Mark your choices with an X. (*Hint:* See Application of Heat and Cold, on pages 590 and 592 in your textbook. Also refer to Chapter 32 in your textbook.)

_____ a. Application of heat

_____ b. Application of cold

_____ c. Elevation of the leg and knee

_____ d. Distraction with a book, TV, or visitor

_____ e. Loud, lively music

_____ f. Favorite music softly played

_____ g. Imagery exercise

_____ h. Relaxation exercise

_____ i. Chiropractic manipulation

➤ • Click on **Exit EPR**. Now click on **Chart** and then on **404**.
  • Select the **Nursing Admission** tab and review this record.

12. Does Clarence Hughes have any particular spiritual beliefs or practices? If so, what are they?

13. Does Clarence Hughes indicate that he has good coping skills?

14. Does he have any special cultural practices?

It is always important to perform an assessment of spirituality, coping ability, and cultural preferences when a patient is admitted. What the assessment reveals should be woven into the plan of care.

Clarence Hughes doesn't have trouble sleeping at home, but in the hospital he finds uninterrupted sleep difficult. The physician has ordered medication to help him sleep.

➤ • Click on **Return to Room 404** and then on **MAR**. Find the medication prescribed for sleep.

15. The physician has ordered _____ to help Clarence Hughes sleep. This

drug should be given _____ before time to sleep. This drug is classified

as a _____. (*Hint:* Use the Drug Guide on the CD-ROM.)

Exercise 2

 CD-ROM Activity—Chronic Pain

 15 minutes

- Sign in to work at Pacific View Regional Hospital on the Medical-Surgical Floor for Period of Care 1. (*Note:* If you are already in the virtual hospital from a previous exercise, click on **Leave the Floor** and then **Restart the Program** to get to the sign-in window.)
- From the Patient List, select Pablo Rodriguez (Room 405).
- Click on **Get Report** and read the note.
- Click on **Go to Nurses' Station**.
- Click on Room **405**.
- Click on **Take Vital Signs** and record them below.

1. Pablo Rodriguez has metastatic carcinoma of the lung and has been admitted with nausea, vomiting, dehydration, and poor pain control. His vital signs at this time are:

BP _____ SpO$_2$ _____ T _____ HR _____ RR _____ Pain level _____

2. What type of pain do you think Pablo Rodriguez is experiencing? (*Hint:* See page 587 in your textbook).

→ • Click on **MAR** and note the medications Pablo Rodriguez is receiving.

3. What is ordered for pain management for Pablo Rodriguez?

4. Pablo Rodriguez is receiving _____ IV as an adjunctive medication to help control his pain.

→ • Click on **Return to Room 405** and then on the **Drug** icon in the lower left corner of the screen.
- Scroll to the medication you listed in question 4.

5. How do you think this medication helps decrease pain?

➔ • Click on **Return to Room 405** and then click on **Chart**.
  • Select the tab for **Nursing Admission** and scroll to the sections on spiritual, cultural, and coping assessment.

6. What does Pablo Rodriguez say about his coping ability?

7. Where does he say his pain is located? How does he describe his pain?

8. Pablo Rodriguez's spiritual orientation is _____, and he feels that

_____.

9. If Pablo Rodriguez were able to take PO medications, what other type of adjunctive medications might help with his pain control? (*Hint:* See page 587 in your textbook).

10. Listed below are interventions used to help relieve pain. Match each specific intervention with its type of measure or therapy. (*Hint:* See Chapter 32 in your textbook).

Intervention	Type of Measure or Therapy
_____ Reposition every hour	a. Adjunctive measure
_____ Keep lights low	b. Comfort measure
_____ Acupuncture	c. Complementary or alternative therapy
_____ Tricyclic antidepressants	
_____ Relaxation exercises	
_____ Imagery exercises	
_____ Change bed linens	
_____ Biofeedback	
_____ Soft music	
_____ Aromatherapy	

→ • Scroll to the Rest and Activity section of the nursing assessment.

11. To help Pablo Rodriguez sleep, you would make sure that there are

    _____ available to help him get comfortable.

12. Is there a sleeping medication ordered for Pablo Rodriguez? (*Hint:* Check the MAR.)

Exercise 3

CD-ROM Activity—Factors that Influence Perception of Pain

20 minutes

- Sign in to work at Pacific View Regional Hospital on the Skilled Nursing Floor for Period of Care 2. (*Note:* If you are already in the virtual hospital from a previous exercise, click on **Leave the Floor** and then **Restart the Program** to get to the sign-in window.)
- From the Patient List, select Kathryn Doyle (Room 503).
- Click on **Get Report**.
- Click on **Go to Nurses' Station**.
- Click on **EPR** and then on **Login**.
- Select **503** in the Patient box. Choose **Vital Signs** in the Category box and scroll backward in time through the vital signs findings.

    1. Kathryn Doyle's pain has ranged from _____ to _____ on a scale of 1-10.

→ • Click on **Exit EPR** and then on Room **503**.
- Click on **Patient Care** and then on **Nurse-Client Interactions**.
- Select and view the video titled **1130: The Unexpected Event**. (*Note:* Check the virtual clock to see whether enough time has elapsed. You can use the fast forward feature to advance the time by two-minute intervals if the video is not yet available. Then click on **Patient Care** and **Nurse-Client Interactions** to refresh the screen.)

    2. What does Kathryn Doyle seem to be experiencing related to this interaction and the events that have occurred?

3. Which of the following factors do you think might make the perception of pain worse? Mark your choices with an X.

_____ a. Pleasant visitors

_____ b. Fear

_____ c. Excessive noise

_____ d. Clean, quiet environment

_____ e. Anxiety

_____ f. Stress

_____ g. Inadequate sleep

_____ h. Attentive nurse

_____ i. Constipation

→ • Click on **MAR** and note the medications ordered for Kathryn Doyle.

4. What medication is ordered for pain for Kathryn Doyle?

5. Is there an adjunctive medication ordered that will help relieve her pain?

6. Oxycodone tends to be constipating. What dietary recommendations would you make to help prevent Kathryn Doyle from experiencing constipation?

7. Kathryn Doyle has _____ ordered to help prevent constipation. (*Hint:* See the MAR.)

8. How does this medication work to help prevent constipation? (*Hint:* Click on the **Drug** icon and read about this drug.)

→ • Click on **EPR** and then on **Login**. Select **503** in the Patient box. Use the Category drop-down menu to select **Gastrointestinal**.

10. Kathryn Doyle had her last bowel movement _____ and

    _____ (is/is not) experiencing constipation.

11. Does Kathryn Doyle have anything ordered to help her sleep? If so, what?

→ • Click on **Exit EPR** and then on **Chart**.
  • Select the chart for **503** and click on the **Nursing Admission** tab. Scroll down to the section on Rest and Activity.

12. What does Kathryn Doyle do in preparation for sleep?

13. How might this activity interfere with her ability to sleep? (*Hint:* Use critical thinking for this question.)

Preparing to Administer Medications

Reading Assignment: Pharmacology and Preparation for Drug Administration
(Chapter 33)
Administering Oral, Topical, and Inhalant Medications
(Chapter 34)

Patients: Jacquline Catanazaro, Medical-Surgical Floor, Room 402
Harry George, Medical-Surgical Floor, Room 401

Objectives:

- Give the rationale for why a patient is receiving a particular drug.
- Calculate drug dosages accurately.
- Identify the nursing implications for drugs a patient is to receive.
- Describe the correct steps for administration of medications.

It is rare that a patient does not have some medication prescribed as part of medical therapy. Medications have a target effect and various side effects. Administering medications safely requires a broad pharmacology knowledge base and adherence to a standard set of steps to prevent errors. Always follow the "five rights" of drug administration: the right drug, the right dose, the right time, the right route, and the right patient. The right drug requires that you understand the action of the drug and why the patient is receiving it. The right dose requires not only that you give exactly the dose ordered, but also that you ensure the ordered dose is within the safe range of the drug for the particular patient. The right time requires that the drug be given at the time it is ordered, and no more than 15 minutes before or 15 minutes after the time. (Some hospitals allow a 30-minute time difference.) This is important so that the patient maintains a steady blood level of the drug. You must also ensure that the drug is within its "use by" date and has not "expired." The right route requires that you give the drug only by the route indicated in the order. If the route needs to be changed, you must contact the physician and have the order changed. To verify that the drug is being given to the right patient, you must verify that the name and ID number on the patient's hospital bracelet matches the imprinted stamp on the Medication Administration Record (MAR). A second check for the right patient is performed by asking the patient to state his or her name. Two separate identifiers must be used *each time* medications are administered. Patient identification is performed before beginning to administer drugs at the bedside. Each of these checks should be performed without distractions and with your full attention.

When preparing medications, you should check each medication for the first four rights three separate times. A good routine is to initially check the medication against the MAR order as you remove it from the patient's medication drawer. Once you have pulled from the drawer all the medications to be given at the time for which you are preparing, perform the second check for each medication. The third check should be done at the bedside just before you open the unit dose package to administer the drug to the patient. It is wise to tell patients what the drug is and why they are receiving it as you give the drug. If patients say they don't recognize the drug or that they shouldn't be receiving it, stop, go back to the chart, and recheck the original order. If it is not clear why a patient is to receive a drug, call the prescriber. Never just go ahead and give a drug to a patient when there is a question about why the patient is receiving it.

Patient education is an important part of drug administration. Teach your patients about the drugs they are receiving. They must know what side effects to look for when they are at home. They should know what they can expect the drug to do for them. Point out adverse effects that should be reported to the prescriber. Review the dosage schedule with each patient and adjust it to the patient's lifestyle if possible. Well-informed patients tend to be more compliant with a drug regimen.

Exercise 1

 CD-ROM Activity—Medication Knowledge

 30 minutes

- Sign in to work at Pacific View Regional Hospital on the Medical-Surgical Floor for Period of Care 1. (*Note:* If you are already in the virtual hospital from a previous exercise, click on **Leave the Floor** and then **Restart the Program** to get to the sign-in window.)
- From the Patient List, select Jacquline Catanazaro (Room 402).
- Click on **Get Report** and read the note.
- Click on **Go to Nurses' Station**.
- Click on **Chart** and then on **402**. Select the tab for **History and Physical** and review.

1. What diagnoses/problems does Jacquline Catanazaro have according to the physician's History and Physical?

- Click on **Return to Nurses' Station**, and then on **MAR**. Select tab **402** and find the medications requested in question 2.
- Again, click on **Return to Nurses' Station**. To complete question 2, consult the Drug Guide by clicking on the **Drug** icon in the lower left corner of your screen.

2. List the oral and topical medications ordered on Jacquline Catanazaro's MAR. For each medication, provide the reason she is receiving it.

Medication	**Reason for Receiving Medication**

3. Match each medication Jacquline Catanazaro is receiving with its classification or mechanism of action.

Medication	**Classification**
_____ Prednisone	a. Antipsychotic-antidepressant
_____ Amoxicillin	b. Non-steroidal antiinflammatory
_____ Ziprasidone	c. Antipsychotic
_____ Ibuprofen	d. Antibiotic-Penicillin
_____ Albuterol	e. Corticosteroid-systemic
_____ Beclomethasone	f. Bronchodilator/antiasthmatic
_____ Ipratropium bromide	g. Adrenocorticosteroid-antiinflammatory
	h. Anticholinergic/bronchodilator

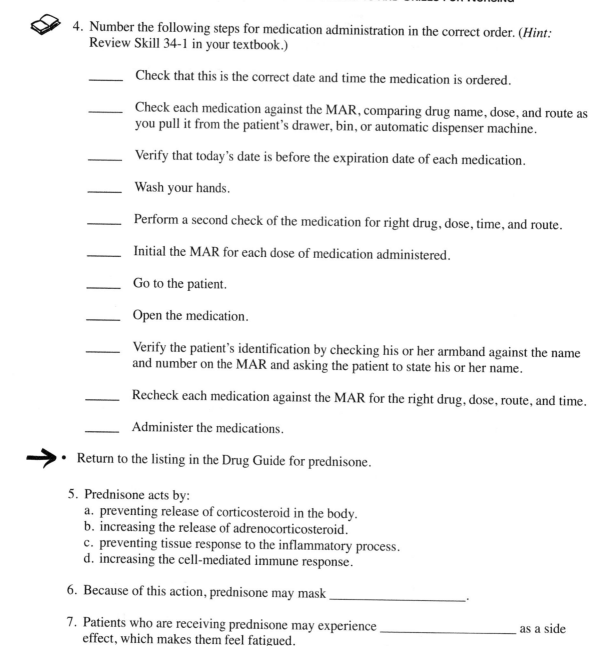

4. Number the following steps for medication administration in the correct order. (*Hint:* Review Skill 34-1 in your textbook.)

_____ Check that this is the correct date and time the medication is ordered.

_____ Check each medication against the MAR, comparing drug name, dose, and route as you pull it from the patient's drawer, bin, or automatic dispenser machine.

_____ Verify that today's date is before the expiration date of each medication.

_____ Wash your hands.

_____ Perform a second check of the medication for right drug, dose, time, and route.

_____ Initial the MAR for each dose of medication administered.

_____ Go to the patient.

_____ Open the medication.

_____ Verify the patient's identification by checking his or her armband against the name and number on the MAR and asking the patient to state his or her name.

_____ Recheck each medication against the MAR for the right drug, dose, route, and time.

_____ Administer the medications.

→ • Return to the listing in the Drug Guide for prednisone.

5. Prednisone acts by:
   a. preventing release of corticosteroid in the body.
   b. increasing the release of adrenocorticosteroid.
   c. preventing tissue response to the inflammatory process.
   d. increasing the cell-mediated immune response.

6. Because of this action, prednisone may mask _____.

7. Patients who are receiving prednisone may experience _____ as a side effect, which makes them feel fatigued.

8. A bone disorder that occurs with long-term prednisone use is _____.

9. When a patient is receiving prednisone, the nurse must do appropriate teaching. Mark with an X those points you would cover in a teaching plan.

_____ a. Single daily dose should be taken before 9:00 a.m.

_____ b. Take it only on an empty stomach, an hour before a meal.

_____ c. Report any other signs of infection.

_____ d. It is okay to have an occasional glass of wine while taking prednisone.

_____ e. Caffeine intake should be limited.

_____ f. Report weight loss promptly.

_____ g. Mood swings are not uncommon.

_____ h. Do not stop taking the drug abruptly.

10. When teaching Jacquline Catanazaro the proper use of her MDI of albuterol, you should instruct her to do the following steps in the correct order. Number these steps in the correct order. (*Hint:* See page 653 in your textbook.)

_____ Wait 1 minute between puffs when more than one puff is ordered.

_____ Place the mouthpiece 1-2 inches in front of the mouth.

_____ Sit or stand up to use the inhaler.

_____ Press the canister down while inhaling.

_____ Shake the canister several times before beginning.

_____ Breathe out through the mouth, emptying the lungs.

_____ Use a bronchodilator MDI before a steroid MDI.

→ • Scroll to find amoxicillin in the Drug Guide.

11. Are there any drug interactions between amoxicillin and the other drugs Jacquline Catanazaro is taking? If so, what are they?

12. If Jacquline Catanazaro, or any patient, has an allergy to _____ or

_____, do not give amoxicillin. Consult the physician in this case.

13. What are the common GI side effects of amoxicillin?

14. For the dose of amoxicillin ordered to be given at 1500, what would you do to try to prevent the GI side effects?

Exercise 2

 CD-ROM Activity—More Medications

 30 minutes

- Sign in to work at Pacific View Regional Hospital on the Medical-Surgical Floor for Period of Care 1. (*Note:* If you are already in the virtual hospital from a previous exercise, click on **Leave the Floor** and then **Restart the Program** to get to the sign-in window.)
- From the Patient List, select Harry George (Room 401).
- Click on **Get Report** and read the note.
- Click on **Go to Nurses' Station**.
- Click on **401** to visit the patient's room.
- Inside the room, click on **Check Allergies**.
- Now click on **Chart** and then on **401**; select the tab for **History and Physical**. Read about Harry George.

1. What are Harry George's diagnoses and/or problems?

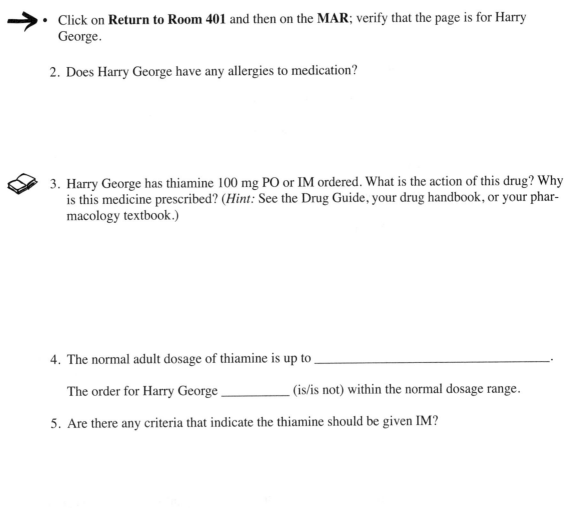

➡ • Click on **Return to Room 401** and then on the **MAR**; verify that the page is for Harry George.

2. Does Harry George have any allergies to medication?

3. Harry George has thiamine 100 mg PO or IM ordered. What is the action of this drug? Why is this medicine prescribed? (*Hint:* See the Drug Guide, your drug handbook, or your pharmacology textbook.)

4. The normal adult dosage of thiamine is up to _____.

The order for Harry George _____ (is/is not) within the normal dosage range.

5. Are there any criteria that indicate the thiamine should be given IM?

➡ • Click on **Return to Room 401**.
   • Click on the **Drug** icon and scroll to Gentamicin. Read about this drug.

6. Although you are not giving Harry George his intravenous medications, you must adhere to the nursing implications for the drugs your patients are receiving. Harry George is receiving gentamicin every 8 hours. This drug has a narrow therapeutic range. A random specimen for drug level is often ordered 8-14 hours after the drug was begun to detect toxic levels and to determine whether the blood level of the drug is within therapeutic range. You should learn both the therapeutic and toxic levels so that you can properly evaluate the laboratory results. If a random specimen was ordered, you should look for laboratory results before the next dose of the drug is administered. What is the toxic level for gentamicin?

7. There are many nursing implications for gentamicin. Which of the following actions are the most important? Mark your choices with an X.

_____ a. Monitor intake and output.

_____ b. Administer the drug between meals.

_____ c. Ask the patient about ringing in the ears or decreased hearing.

_____ d. Administer the drug only with a meal.

_____ e. Report nausea promptly.

_____ f. Give IM injection quickly.

_____ g. Do not give if patient is dehydrated.

_____ h. Assess for skin rash.

_____ i. Report diarrhea promptly.

8. Are there any drug interactions between gentamicin and the other drugs Harry George is receiving? (*Hint:* Read the Interactions section of the entry for gentamicin in the Drug Guide.)

9. Harry George has trimethobenzamide HCl 250 mg (Tigan) PO ordered q6h prn nausea and

   vomiting. Trimethobenzamide HCl is an _____ class drug. (*Hint:* Scroll through the Drug Guide and read about this drug.)

10. Harry George is also receiving chlordiazepoxide HCl, and hydromorphone. What is the potential interaction effect of these drugs with trimethobenzamide HCl? (*Hint:* Check the Drug Guide for the class and action of each of these two drugs.)

11. Harry George has glyburide ordered to help treat his diabetes. What is the mechanism of action of this drug? (*Hint:* Check the Drug Guide.)

12. What type or class of drug is glyburide?

13. Glyburide begins working within _____ to _____ minutes.

14. The glyburide is listed on the MAR to be given at 0800. What would you want to know before administering the drug at that time? (*Hint:* See your pharmacology book or your nursing drug handbook.)

We will look at the parenteral drugs Harry George is receiving in another lesson.

15. Below, list the PO and topical drugs that are ordered for Harry George. For each drug, provide its action or the reason for administration.

Medication	**Action and/or Reason for Administration**

Oral Medication Administration

Reading Assignment: Pharmacology and Preparation for Drug Administration
(Chapter 33)
Administering Oral, Topical, and Inhalant Medications
(Chapter 34)

Patients: Harry George, Medical-Surgical Floor, Room 401

Clarence Hughes, Medical-Surgical Floor, Room 404

Objectives:

- Safely administer oral medications.
- Identify the nursing assessments necessary before administering a drug.
- Know the potential side effects and adverse effects of the drugs being administered.
- Identify any interactions between drugs being administered and other drugs that patient is taking.

All medication orders are to be checked and verified with the MAR at least every 24 hours. The nurse must be alert to when each patient's other health care providers are on the unit and check to see whether new medication orders have been written. The five rights and five responsibilities should be followed *each* time that medications are administered to *each* patient. When preparing to administer medications, distractions should be reduced as much as possible. Do not talk with others while preparing medications. Always use at least two identifiers when checking for the right patient. If the patient questions any medication or does not understand why it is prescribed, stop and reverify the order. Call the prescriber if necessary. Continue teaching your patients about their medications each time you administer them. Assess whether the patient is compliant with medication regimens when at home.

Check the Laboratory Reports section of the patient's chart to ascertain lab values that are pertinent to the medication you are about to give. When giving antibiotics, assess the patient and the lab values to see whether the medication is what is indicated for the disorder and whether medications already given have been effective.

Check for patient allergies by looking at the MAR, the chart cover, and the Nursing Admission—and by asking the patient. This is especially important for every antibiotic you are about to administer.

Exercise 1

 CD-ROM Activity—Administering PO Medications

 45 minutes

- Sign in to work at Pacific View Regional Hospital on the Medical-Surgical Floor for Period of Care 1. (*Note:* If you are already in the virtual hospital from a previous exercise, click on **Leave the Floor** and then **Restart the Program** to get to the sign-in window.)
- From the Patient List, select Harry George (Room 401).
- Click on **Get Report** and review the information about this patient.
- Click on **Go to Nurses' Station** and then on **401**.
- Click on **Patient Care** and then on **Medication Administration**.
- Prepare to give Harry George his 0800 PO medications. (*Hint:* First click on **MAR** and find his orders.)

1. Which oral medications is Harry George scheduled to receive at 0800 according to his MAR?

2. Are there any assessments that you need to make before preparing and administering these medications? (*Hint:* Harry George is diabetic, so you might want to know his morning blood glucose determination. Click on **Return to Room 401** and then on **Chart**. Select the chart for **401** and click on **Nurse's Notes**.) What was the blood glucose?

3. Mark with an X each of the system assessments you should make before giving the 0800 PO medications.

   _____ a. Chest

   _____ b. Abdomen

   _____ c. Head & Neck

   _____ d. Upper Extremities

   _____ e. Lower Extremities

   _____ f. Back & Spine

→ • Click on **Return to Room 401**.

• Now click on **Medication Room** and prepare Harry George's 0800 medications.

• Click on **Unit Dosage** or on the unit dose cart and then on drawer **401** to access Harry George's medications.

• Highlight the correct drug to be removed from the drawer by clicking on it.

• Verify the MAR order with the medication information on dosage and route on the unit dose label (shown on the right side of the screen).

• Click on **Put Medication on Tray**.

• After each medication has been moved to the tray, click on **Review Your Medications** and reverify the drug, dosage, and route compared with the MAR information. This is your second check of the medication after removing it from the drawer.

• After your review of each medication, click on **Close Drawer** in the lower right corner of the screen and then click on **View Medication Room**.

• Now click on **Preparation** or on the tray sitting on the counter on the left side of your screen. Verify the drug label with the order and click **Prepare**. This activates the Preparation Wizard. Supply any requested information; then click **Next**.

• Click on the correct patient's room number and name and then click on **Finish**.

4. Below, document the medications ordered for Harry George at 0800.

Medication Order	Route	To Be Administered By You?

5. Harry George's medical record number is _____.

6. Does the medication label tell you the medication expiration date?

7. Glyburide can increase the activity of oral _____. (*Hint:* Consult the Drug Guide or your drug handbook.)

8. Is Harry George receiving the above-mentioned drug?

- Click on **Return to Medication Room** and then on **401**.
- Inside the patient's room, click on **Check Armband** to correctly identify Harry George as the patient for whom your medications are intended.
- Now click on **Check Allergies** and review this information.
- Click on **Patient Care** and then on **Medication Administration**. When the tray appears (the list of medications you prepared, shown in the purple box on the left side of the screen), click on the down arrow next to **Select**.
- Click on **Administer**. Choose the correct route from the drop-down menu. Next, select the correct method from the drop-down menu.
- Once you are sure everything has been checked three times and that the medication meets the order criteria and the correct time, click on **Administer to Patient**. Document that you have given the drug by clicking on **Yes**. Repeat this process for each medication on your tray. Finally, click **Finish**.

9. What, if any, allergy does Harry George have?

10. Glyburide peaks in _____ and lasts _____ hours.

11. Why is it important that Harry George eat his meals when he is taking this medication?

12. Patients with diabetes can become hypoglycemic or hyperglycemic for a variety of reasons. It is important that the nurse know whether this is happening. Below, match each sign or symptom with the correct disorder. (*Hint:* See your textbook for the signs of hypo- and hyperglycemia or check the Drug Guide. It is important to memorize these signs and symptoms.)

Sign or Symptom	**Disorder**
_____ Blurred vision	a. Hyperglycemia
_____ Thirst	b. Hypoglycemia
_____ Shakiness or tremors	
_____ Rapid respirations	
_____ Headache	
_____ Tachycardia	
_____ Hunger	
_____ Cool, clammy skin	
_____ Nausea or vomiting	
_____ Increased urination	

• Click on **Leave the Floor** and then select **Look at Your Preceptor's Evaluation**. Click on **Medication Scorecard** to see how you did with the medication administration for Harry George.

Exercise 2

 CD-ROM Activity—Administering More Medications

 30 minutes

- Sign in to work at Pacific View Regional Hospital on the Medical-Surgical Floor for Period of Care 1. (*Note:* If you are already in the virtual hospital from a previous exercise, click on **Leave the Floor** and then **Restart the Program** to get to the sign-in window.)
- From the Patient List, select Clarence Hughes (Room 404).
- Click on **Get Report** and review the information.
- Click on **Go to Nurses' Station**.
- Click on **MAR** and note the medications to be administered to Clarence Hughes at 0800. (*Hint:* You will need to record these orders in the table in question 2.)
- Click on **Return to Nurses' Station** and then on **404** to go to the patient's room.
- Click on **Clinical Alerts** and determine what assessments need to be made before you administer medications. (*Hint:* You will use this information to answer question 5.)

1. What is the first thing you should do before going to the Medication Room and pulling medications for patients from the drawers or bins?

2. Below, copy the orders for the oral 0800 medications, as well as any PRN medications, to be given to Clarence Hughes. (*Hint:* Use the Drug Guide to determine classification.)

Medication Order	Route	Classification of Medication

3. Clarence Hughes' hospital number is _____.

4. What does a valid medication order contain? (*Hint:* See page 617 in your textbook.)

5. Based on your review of the **Clinical Alerts** what assessments should you perform? (*Hint:* Click on **Patient Care** and then on the areas of assessment necessary.)

→ • Click on **Check Allergies**.

6. Does Clarence Hughes have any drug allergies?

7. Is the order on the MAR for oxycodone with acetaminophen a valid order? If not, what is missing?

8. What would you do before giving the oxycodone with acetaminophen?

- Click on **Medication Room** at the bottom of the screen.
- Click on **Unit Dosage** or on the unit dosage cart and then on drawer **404**.
- Click on the first medication you wish to administer to Clarence Hughes at 0800. Verify the unit dose medication label with the order as you take it from the drawer, following the five rights.
- Click on **Put Medication on Tray**. Continue this process for each medication that you are going to administer.
- Click on **Close Drawer** and then on **View Medication Room** in the lower right corner.
- Click on **Automated System** to obtain the controlled drug. Click **Login**.
- Select **Clarence Hughes, 404**. Choose the correct drawer for the medication you want. (Assume the order is for the 5/325 dosage.) Click **Open Drawer**.
- Select the correct medication and click on **Put Medication on Tray**. Then click on **Close Drawer**.
- Click on **Review Your Medications**. Highlight each medication in turn and perform your second medication check with the drug order. Use the five rights!
- Click on **Return to Medication Room** and then on **View Medication Room**.

9. What do you need to do before you prepare the medications you have put on the tray?

- Click on **Preparation** or on the tray on the counter on the left side of the screen.
- Click on **Prepare** and then supply any information requested by the Preparation Wizard before clicking **Finish**. Continue this process for each medication.
- Click on **Return to Medication Room**.
- Click on **404** to return to Clarence Hughes' room.

10. You have just entered Clarence Hughes' room. What should you do at this point?

11. When and how do you perform your third check of the medications?

- Click on **Patient Care** and then on **Medication Administration**.
- Follow the steps in the Administration Wizard until you have administered all the medications you prepared. (*Hint:* If you need help with any of these steps, refer to pages 26-30 and 36-40 in the **Getting Started** section of this workbook.)

12. What do you need to do after you have administered all of the medications for this time period?

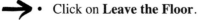

- Click on **Leave the Floor**.
- Click on **Look at Your Preceptor's Evaluation**. Click on **Medication Scorecard** and review the evaluation.

18

Administering Injections and Topical Medications

⁄☞ Reading Assignment: Administering Oral, Topical, and Inhalant Medications (Chapter 34)

Administering Intradermal, Subcutaneous, and Intramuscular Injections (Chapter 35)

Patients: Harry George, Medical-Surgical Floor, Room 401

Clarence Hughes, Medical-Surgical Floor, Room 404

Patricia Newman, Medical-Surgical Floor, Room 406

Objectives:

- Correctly administer subcutaneous injections.
- Identify injection sites for intramuscular injections.
- Correctly administer an intramuscular injection.
- Safely administer ophthalmic medications.
- Use correct technique when applying a medicated skin patch.

Every nurse must know the sites where subcutaneous and intramuscular injections can be administered. When heparin or insulin is given on an ongoing basis, the sites must be rotated. Thus it is important to document the location in which each injection was given. Check the MAR, the Nurse's Notes, or flow sheet to see where the previous injection was given before deciding on which site to use.

Dangerous drugs such as insulin, heparin, and cardiac injectable drugs should be double-checked by another nurse before they are administered. The other nurse should verify that you have interpreted the order correctly and that you have calculated the dose properly and drawn up the correct amount of the drug.

Ophthalmic drops and ointments must be kept sterile and must be applied correctly in order to achieve their intended effect. Patients must be taught how to correctly use these medications.

Medications that are prescribed in slow-release skin patches must be applied properly, and old patches must be removed when a new one is applied. Each year more drugs are available in this form. It is easy to miss a skin patch under a patient gown or pajamas. If that happens, the patient may receive more of the drug than is prescribed.

Exercise 1

 CD-ROM Activity—Administering Insulin

 30 minutes

- Sign in to work at Pacific View Regional Hospital on the Medical-Surgical Floor for Period of Care 1. (*Note:* If you are already in the virtual hospital from a previous exercise, click on **Leave the Floor** and then **Restart the Program** to get to the sign-in window.)
- From the Patient List, select Harry George (Room 401).
- Click on **Get Report** and review the information.
- Click on **Go to Nurses' Station**.
- Click on Room **401** to visit Harry George. Let's assume that when you ask the patient how he is feeling, he tells you that he is a little nauseous.
- Click on **MAR** to see what medication is ordered that may help relieve the nausea.
- Click on **Return to 401** and visit Harry George to see whether he needs anything else before you prepare this medication.

1. Harry George's MAR indicates he is to receive thiamine 100 mg once a day. What is the maximum safe dose for an adult? Assume that you need to give this medication IM today. (*Hint:* Use the Drug Guide to find thiamine and read about this drug. Note that normally you would administer this drug along with his other oral medications.)

→ • Click on **Medication Room** and then on **Unit Dosage**. Choose the drawer for **401**.
- Click on the correct drug to be removed from the drawer.
- Verify the MAR order with the dosage and route information on the unit dosage label.
- Click on **Put Medication on Tray**.
- Perform your second check of the medication by clicking on **Review Your Medications**. Reverify the drug, dosage, and route—and that it is intended to be given at this time on this date.
- Click on **Return to Medication Room**, then on **Close Drawer**, and then on **View Medication Room**.

2. What size syringe and needle will you choose to give this injection to Harry George?

3. What must you do before beginning to prepare the medications?

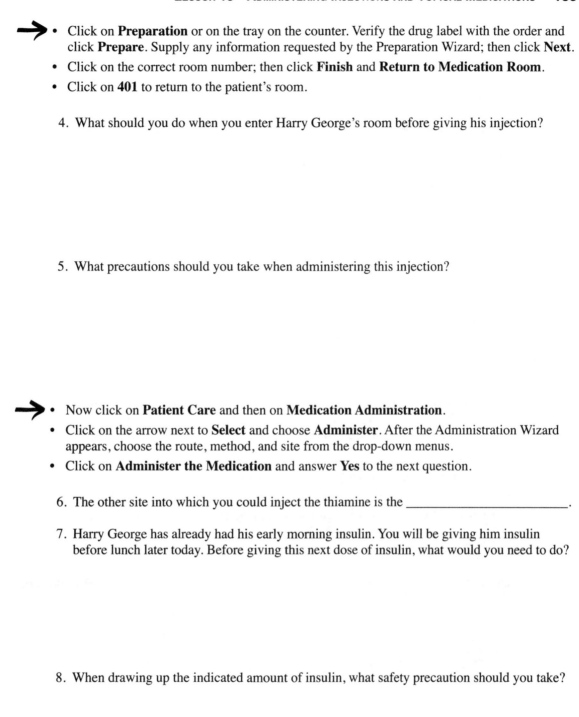

→ • Click on **Preparation** or on the tray on the counter. Verify the drug label with the order and click **Prepare**. Supply any information requested by the Preparation Wizard; then click **Next**.

• Click on the correct room number; then click **Finish** and **Return to Medication Room**.

• Click on **401** to return to the patient's room.

4. What should you do when you enter Harry George's room before giving his injection?

5. What precautions should you take when administering this injection?

→ • Now click on **Patient Care** and then on **Medication Administration**.

• Click on the arrow next to **Select** and choose **Administer**. After the Administration Wizard appears, choose the route, method, and site from the drop-down menus.

• Click on **Administer the Medication** and answer **Yes** to the next question.

6. The other site into which you could inject the thiamine is the _____.

7. Harry George has already had his early morning insulin. You will be giving him insulin before lunch later today. Before giving this next dose of insulin, what would you need to do?

8. When drawing up the indicated amount of insulin, what safety precaution should you take?

9. What must you check on the insulin vial *besides* the name of the drug and the dose per mL?

10. When regular and NPH insulin are ordered to be given together, you would draw up

    the _____ insulin first. (*Hint:* See page 674 in your textbook.)

11. Regular insulin has its onset in _____, peaks in _____,

    and has a duration of _____. (*Hint:* Consult the Drug Guide.)

12. What area is preferred for insulin injection?

Exercise 2

CD-ROM Activity—Heparin Administration and Ophthalmic Medication Administration

30 minutes

- Sign in to work at Pacific View Regional Hospital on the Medical-Surgical Floor for Period of Care 1. (*Note:* If you are already in the virtual hospital from a previous exercise, click on **Leave the Floor** and then **Restart the Program** to get to the sign-in window.)
- From the Patient List, select Clarence Hughes (Room 404).
- Click on **Get Report** and review the information.
- Click on **Go to Nurses' Station**.
- Click on **MAR** and check for the enoxaparin injection that Clarence Hughes is to receive.

1. Complete the table below based on the MAR order for enoxaparin.

Drug Order	Classification	Action	Precautions

2. What is the most likely reason enoxaparin is ordered for Clarence Hughes?

3. Enoxaparin is usually given after knee replacement surgery for an average of

   _____. (*Hint:* Consult the Drug Guide on the CD-ROM.)

4. If Clarence Hughes experienced bleeding problems, you would give the antidote for

   enoxaparin, which is_____.

5. When administering enoxaparin, which of the following would you do to provide Clarence Hughes with the dose ordered? Mark your choices with an X. (*Hint:* See pages 681-683 of your textbook and the listing in the Drug Guide.)

   _____ a. Use any subcutaneous site.

   _____ b. Use the prefilled syringe of 0.3 mL.

   _____ c. Use a 5/8-inch needle at a 45-degree angle.

   _____ d. Use a 1/2-inch needle at a 90-degree angle.

   _____ e. Use a 2-mL syringe.

   _____ f. Use the abdominal area lateral and below the umbilicus.

   _____ g. Pull the tissue taut before introducing the needle.

   _____ h. Pinch up the tissue in a roll before introducing the needle.

   _____ i. Inject deep into the subcutaneous tissue.

   _____ j. Do not aspirate before injecting this medication.

   _____ k. Rub the area gently after injection to hasten absorption.

   _____ l. Wait at least 15 seconds after injecting before withdrawing the needle.

6. What laboratory test would you want to check to see whether this drug is effective? (*Hint:* See your textbook or a pharmacology book.)

→ • Return to Clarence Hughes' MAR and note the ophthalmic solutions ordered for him. Read about these medications in the Drug Guide.

7. Timolol and pilocarpine are used for what disorder?

Read in your medical-surgical textbook about the disorder you identified in question 7.

8. If Clarence Hughes does not use his eye drops, what could be the consequences?

9. If these are new medications for Clarence Hughes, what points of patient teaching should you cover? (*Hint:* Check a pharmacology book or nursing drug handbook.)

Exercise 3

 CD-ROM Activity—Transdermal Medication

 15 minutes

- Sign in to work at Pacific View Regional Hospital on the Medical-Surgical Floor for Period of Care 1. (*Note:* If you are already in the virtual hospital from a previous exercise, click on **Leave the Floor** and then **Restart the Program** to get to the sign-in window.)
- From the Patient List, select Patricia Newman (Room 406).
- Click on **Get Report** and review the information.
- Click on **Go to Nurses' Station**.
- Click on **MAR** and then on tab **406**. Note the transdermal patch ordered for Patricia Newman.

1. Below, list the information for the transdermal patch ordered for Patricia Newman. (*Hint:* Consult a pharmacology book, nursing drug handbook, or the Drug Guide on the CD-ROM.)

Medication Order	Classification	Action/Reason for Administration

2. Was the transdermal skin patch applied on Tuesday? (*Hint:* Go to the chart and check the Expired MARs to see whether the drug was administered.)

3. What should you do with the information you just discovered?

4. Where should a skin patch be placed on the body? (*Hint:* See page 655 in your textbook.)

5. After application, the patch should be _____ for identification of when it was applied. (*Hint:* See page 656 in your textbook.)

6. When applying a new transdermal patch, you should always

_____.

7. What is necessary to do to ensure that the transdermal patch will adhere properly?

19

Caring for Patients Receiving Intravenous Therapy

Reading Assignment: Administering Intravenous Solutions and Medications
(Chapter 36)

Patients: Harry George, Medical-Surgical Floor, Room 401
Piya Jordan, Medical-Surgical Floor, Room 403

Objectives:

- Follow safe practice in the administration of IV fluids.
- Identify signs of IV infiltration.
- List the signs and symptoms of complications of IV therapy.
- Perform assessments essential for the patient receiving IV fluids.
- Monitor patients for side effects of IV medications.

Whether or not you are allowed to hang intravenous solutions or administer IV medications, you should know about the types of solutions that are used, the guidelines related to the use of this route, and how to monitor the rate of flow. Caring for patients undergoing intravenous therapy includes calculating and checking that the flow rate is correct at the beginning of the shift, any time the patient has been up and has returned to bed or the chair, and when you are at the bedside for another reason. Do not assume that because an IV pump is in use that it is functioning properly. Always leave pump alarms turned on. Throughout the shift, track on the IV bag the amount infused over a specific time and determine that the amount is accurate with the flow rate ordered. Assess the patient for signs and symptoms of complications of IV therapy at the beginning of the shift and every 4 hours. Keep IV tubing unkinked and out from under the patient.

When patients are receiving intravenous therapy, they must be assessed carefully for potential local and systemic complications. Infants and older adults are especially susceptible to circulatory overload. Infiltration and phlebitis often occur at the IV site. Speed shock can occur if the flow rate is not carefully controlled.

Know the drugs the patient is receiving intravenously, even though you may not be administering them yourself. IV fluids and medications are made instantly available for circulation to all tissues of the body. Because you are giving a drug or solution directly through a vein into the circulation, all solutions and equipment must be sterile to avoid introducing a source of infection.

When an IV catheter is removed, it should be inspected carefully to determine whether a piece of it has broken off. If a piece of catheter is left in the vein, a catheter embolus can occur.

When a blood product is administered, the patient is monitored particularly closely. Whether you are allowed to hang blood in your state or you are just assisting with monitoring the patient, you should know all of the guidelines for the administration of blood products.

Exercise 1

 CD-ROM Activity—Monitoring the Patient Receiving Intravenous Therapy

 30 minutes

- Sign in to work at Pacific View Regional Hospital on the Medical-Surgical Floor for Period of Care 1. (*Note:* If you are already in the virtual hospital from a previous exercise, click on **Leave the Floor** and then **Restart the Program** to get to the sign-in window.)
- From the Patient List, select Harry George (Room 401).
- Click on **Get Report** and read the note.
- Click on **Go to Nurses' Station** and then click on **Chart**.
- Click on the chart for **401**. Select the tab for **Physician's Orders** and note the solutions and medications Harry George is currently receiving intravenously.

  1. Below, list the intravenous solutions and medications ordered for Harry George. For each medication, give the classification, along with its action or the reason it is ordered.

Medication Order	Classification	Action/Reason for Administration

You should become familiar with the side effects and nursing implications for these drugs since you are caring for Harry George.

2. Name the three most important nursing implications for the benzodiazepine drugs. (*Hint:* Consult a pharmacology book, nursing drug handbook, or the Drug Guide on the CD-ROM.)

   a.

   b.

   c.

→ • Now click on **Return to Nurses' Station** and then on **401**. Inside the patient's room, click on **Patient Care** and then on **Upper Extremities**. Assess Harry George's IV site.

3. Where is Harry George's IV site located?

4. Document your findings concerning the IV site here.

5. What question(s) would you ask Harry George about his IV site?

6. If tubing that delivers 15 drops per mL is being used, the IV will be flowing at _____ drops per minute. (*Hint:* See page 704 in your textbook.)

7. What is the purpose of administering an isotonic intravenous solution? (*Hint:* See page 696 in your textbook.)

→ • Click on **Chart** and then on **401**. Click on the tab for **Nurse's Notes**. Read through the notes.

8. As far as you can tell, when was Harry George's IV cannula inserted?

9. Is the IV cannula due to be changed today? Are there any indications that it should be changed? (*Hint:* Click on the **Emergency Department** tab and read the ED nurse's notes.)

→ • Click on **Return to Room 401**; then click on **EPR** and **Login**. Select **401** as the Patient and **IV** as the category. Highlight the data to see the pertinent abbreviations for interpretation of the documentation.

10. When was the IV tubing last changed? How often should the tubing be changed?

→ • When a patient is receiving intravenous fluid, the nurse should monitor the electrolyte values to determine whether the intravenous therapy is causing any electrolyte imbalance.
  • Click on **Exit EPR** and go to the chart to find the electrolyte lab values. (*Hint:* Click on **Chart**, **401**, and the tab for **Laboratory Reports**.)

11. Harry George's potassium level is _____. His sodium level is _____. His

_____ level is above normal and most likely indicates a state of slight dehydration. The slightly elevated chloride level is consistent with the sodium level.

12. What laboratory report would you check to see whether there is an indication that the antibiotics Harry George is receiving are effective?

Exercise 2

  CD-ROM Activity—Complications of Intravenous Therapy

15 minutes

1. Match each sign or symptom below with its related IV therapy complication.

Sign or Symptom	**Complication of IV Therapy**
_____ Coolness surrounding the IV site	a. Infiltration
_____ Redness at the IV site	b. Phlebitis
_____ Sudden drop in BP with increase in pulse rate	c. Thrombophlebitis
	d. Infection at site
_____ Redness of the vein used for IV therapy	e. Air embolus
_____ Red site with itching and rash	f. Speed shock
_____ Hardness along the vein used for IV therapy	g. Infection
_____ Fever, chills, general malaise	h. Circulatory overload
_____ Flushed face and severe headache	i. Allergic reaction to IV medication
_____ Warmth at the IV site	
_____ IV flow sluggish with redness and tenderness at site	
_____ IV site hot, red, and painful	
_____ Elevated BP, dyspnea, crackles in lungs	

2. What should you do if IV infiltration occurs?

3. If the IV flow has slowed considerably after the patient has been up for a sponge bath, what basic actions would you take before assuming that the cannula is clotted?

4. How often should you check on your patient to assess the IV site and flow rate when IV therapy is in progress?

 5. You are monitoring your patient's IV. It is to run at 100 mL/hr. The tubing the hospital uses delivers 10 drops per mL. How many drops per minute should the IV deliver? (*Hint:* See Table 36-3 in your textbook.)
   a. 16 drops a minute
   b. 21 drops a minute
   c. 28 drops a minute
   d. 25 drops a minute

Exercise 3

 CD-ROM Activity—Monitoring the Patient Receiving a Blood Transfusion

 30 minutes

Piya Jordan has a blood transfusion ordered. As her nurse for the shift, you will be monitoring her, even if you are not allowed to hang blood as a student or LPN/LVN in your state.

• Sign in to work at Pacific View Regional Hospital on the Medical-Surgical Floor for Period of Care 2. (*Note:* If you are already in the virtual hospital from a previous exercise, click on **Leave the Floor** and then **Restart the Program** to get to the sign-in window.)
• From the Patient List, select Piya Jordan (Room 403).
• Click on **Get Report** and read the note.
• Click on **Go to Nurses' Station** and then on **Chart**.
• Click on **403** and select the **Physician's Notes**. Review to find out what blood product is planned for Piya Jordan.

   1. The physician has planned to give Piya Jordan 2 units of _____.

2. Why is Piya Jordan receiving this blood transfusion? What laboratory parameters would you check before the blood is administered so that you will know later whether the transfusion was effective? (*Hint:* See the Laboratory Reports in her chart.)

3. In order for this blood product to be administered, Piya Jordan should have an

   _____ IV cannula in place.

→ • Click on the **Nurse's Notes** tab and read the note for Wednesday at 0745.

4. Is the IV cannula that Piya Jordan has in place the correct size for the blood product transfusion?

5. Is there a valid consent signed by Piya Jordan for the blood transfusion? (*Hint:* Click on **Consents** in the chart.)

6. Which of the following are pertinent guidelines when administering a blood transfusion? Mark your choices with an X. (*Hint:* See pages 718-724 in your textbook.)

   _____ a. Blood must be kept refrigerated until it is administered.

   _____ b. Gloves must be used when discontinuing a blood product transfusion.

   _____ c. Blood products are administered along with D_5W IV solution.

   _____ d. Vital signs must be taken every hour while a blood product is infusing.

   _____ e. Stay with the patient during the first 15 minutes of the infusion.

   _____ f. The infusion should run at 2 mL/min for the first 15 minutes.

   _____ g. Vital signs are taken every 30 minutes if they are stable after the first 15 minutes.

   _____ h. Two nurses must verify the donor number, patient ID number, patient name, and ABO and Rh type on the blood bag, on the patient's blood armband, and on the slip accompanying the unit.

7. The average infusion time for a unit of packed red cells is:
   a. 30 minutes
   b. 1 hour
   c. 2 hours
   d. 4 hours

8. Each patient must be carefully monitored for a transfusion reaction. Signs and symptoms of such a reaction include which of the following? (Mark your choices with an X.)

   _____ a. Chills

   _____ b. Fever

   _____ c. Stomach ache

   _____ d. Back pain

   _____ e. Cramps in the legs

   _____ f. Itching

   _____ g. Shortness of breath

   _____ h. Cough

   _____ i. Feels "funny"

9. What must be done immediately if a patient exhibits signs or symptoms of a transfusion reaction? (*Hint:* See Skill 36-6 on page 723 in your textbook.)

10. Most transfusion reactions occur during _____ of the infusion.

Caring for the Surgical Patient

📖 **Reading Assignment:** Care of the Surgical Patient (Chapter 37)

Patients: Piya Jordan, Medical-Surgical Floor, Room 403
Clarence Hughes, Medical-Surgical Floor, Room 404

Objectives:

- Identify preoperative procedures necessary for the patient scheduled for surgery.
- List measures to be carried out for the patient to be readied for surgery.
- Discuss care in the postanesthesia care unit (PACU).
- Identify necessary elements of the PACU report to the floor.

The surgical experience may produce a great deal of anxiety in the patient. Today, patients who are not already in the hospital must arrive at the hospital in the very early hours the morning before surgery. This means they are awake long before their normal waking time. Preoperative care is provided quickly and efficiently, but often there is not sufficient time for teaching about what to expect or explaining about postoperative care.

During surgery, the circulating nurse and the operating team watch out for the patient's welfare. After surgery, the patient's care is transferred to the PACU nurse for a short period of time. When the patient is stable, transfer to the surgical floor occurs. "Same-day-surgery" patients who have had more minor surgical procedures are discharged to home.

Exercise 1

 CD-ROM Activity—Preoperative Care

 30 minutes

- Sign in to work at Pacific View Regional Hospital on the Medical-Surgical Floor for Period of Care 1. (*Note:* If you are already in the virtual hospital from a previous exercise, click on **Leave the Floor** and then **Restart the Program** to get to the sign-in window.)
- From the Patient List, select Piya Jordan (Room 403).
- Click on **Get Report** and read the note.
- Click on **Go to Nurses' Station**.
- Click on **Chart** and then on **403**.
- Click on the **Surgical Reports** tab. Scroll to the Preoperative Patient Instruction Sheet.

1. What instructions regarding hygiene were given to Piya Jordan in preparation for her surgery?

2. What were the instructions regarding eating or drinking?

3. According to the surgical admission sheet, Piya Jordan was scheduled for a

   _____.

Read in your medical-surgical textbook about colectomy.

4. What does a colectomy involve? Why is it being done in Piya Jordan's case? (*Hint:* Click on the **History and Physical** tab and review.)

5. Which of the following risk factors for surgical complications apply to Piya Jordan? Mark your choices with an X. (*Hint:* Continue reviewing the History and Physical.)

   _____ a. Obesity

   _____ b. Age

   _____ c. Blood disorder

   _____ d. Heart disease

   _____ e. Respiratory disease

   _____ f. Immune disorder

   _____ g. Drug abuse

   _____ h. Chronic pain

→ • Return to the **Surgical Reports** section of the chart. Scroll to the Surgery Procedures and Treatments form.

6. The preoperative sedation Piya Jordan received was _____.

Read in your pharmacology book or your nursing drug handbook about this medication.

7. Below, provide the requested information about the preoperative medication you provided in question 6.

Medication Order	Action	Onset and Duration

8. Before administering preoperative medications, what must be checked or done? (*Hint:* See pages 736-737 in your textbook.)

9. When the nurse was teaching Piya Jordan about the use of the incentive spirometer preoperatively, she should have told her to do what? (*Hint:* See page 517 in your textbook.)
   a. Inhale through her nose.
   b. Complete five full breaths for each session.
   c. Inhale completely and hold for at least 3 seconds.
   d. Exhale completely and hold for at least 10 seconds.

10. From the following list, identify the tubes and devices that Piya Jordan was told will be in place postoperatively. Mark your choices with an X. (*Hint:* Review the preoperative surgical report forms in the chart.)

   _____ a. Abdominal binder

   _____ b. IV

   _____ c. NG tube

   _____ d. Foley catheter

   _____ e. Sequential compression devices (SCDs)

   _____ f. Abduction wedge

   _____ g. Patient analgesia controller

   _____ h. J-P suction device with drain

   _____ i. Traction apparatus

Exercise 2

Writing Activity—Intraoperative and Postanesthesia Care

15 minutes

1. Piya Jordan received _____ anesthesia.

2. The roles of the scrub nurse and the circulating nurse vary. Identify which functions each nurse would perform for Piya Jordan by matching the functions with the appropriate nurse or nurses. (*Hint:* See pages 742-743 in your textbook.)

Functions	**Nurse**
_____ Sets up the instruments	a. Circulating nurse
_____ Carries out the "time out" surgical site identification	b. Scrub nurse
_____ Gowns and gloves the surgeon	c. Circulating and scrub nurse
_____ Points out breaks in sterile technique	
_____ Counts sponges and instruments	
_____ Hands instruments to the operating team	
_____ Obtains needed fluids and medications	
_____ Takes charge of tissue specimens	
_____ Positions lights and stools	
_____ Assists with gowning and gloving	
_____ Checks function of each piece of equipment	
_____ Verifies that the electric cautery is properly grounded	
_____ Positions patient on the table and pads potential pressure areas	
_____ Communicates with those outside the OR	

3. The _____ monitors the patient's vital signs during the operation.

4. When surgery is over, the patient is moved to the postanesthesia care unit (PACU) and

is positioned to _____ and

_____. (*Hint:* See page 743 in your textbook.)

5. In the PACU, the vital signs are measured and documented _____ until

_____.

6. The Aldrete scoring system is often used to determine when the patient is ready for transfer back to the nursing unit. Mark with an X each area that is scored with this system. (*Hint:* See pages 743-744 in your textbook.)

_____ a. Time in PACU

_____ b. Respiration

_____ c. Consciousness

_____ d. Gag reflex

_____ e. Skin color

_____ f. Circulation

_____ g. Activity

_____ h. Speech

7. Two important functions of the PACU nurse are to keep the patient _____

and to reassure the patient that _____.

8. Because Piya Jordan has preexisting atrial fibrillation, the PACU nurse will monitor her closely. What assessments should the nurse perform related to this problem? (*Hint:* Use critical thinking for this question.)

Exercise 3

 CD-ROM Activity—Another Surgery

 30 minutes

- Sign in to work at Pacific View Regional Hospital on the Medical-Surgical Floor for Period of Care 1. (*Note:* If you are already in the virtual hospital from a previous exercise, click on **Leave the Floor** and then **Restart the Program** to get to the sign-in window.)
- From the Patient List, select Clarence Hughes (Room 404).
- Click on **Get Report** and read the note.
- Click on **Go to Nurses' Station** then on **404** to visit Clarence Hughes.
- Click on **Chart** and then on the chart for **404**. Click on the tab for **Surgical Reports**.

1. The surgical procedure that Clarence Hughes underwent was a _____

   _____ .

2. Preoperatively, the nurse verifies the disposition of Clarence Hughes' valuables. What does the preoperative form indicate as to the disposition of his valuables?

3. How would you handle it if a patient did not want to remove his or her wedding ring? (*Hint:* See page 736 in your textbook.)

4. Because of the type of surgery Clarence Hughes had, he will not be able to exercise his foot and leg to the same extent that Piya Jordan is encouraged to do postoperatively. He is at high risk for deep vein thrombosis. What would you encourage him to do with the lower left extremity? (*Hint:* See Patient Teaching 37-1 on page 733 in your textbook.)

5. What scheduled medications did the surgeon OK for Clarence Hughes to have in the immediate preoperative period? (*Hint:* Review the Surgical Reports section of the chart.)

6. Below, note the preoperative medication that Clarence Hughes received, along with the action, onset, and duration of each. (*Hint:* See the Drug Guide or check your pharmacology or nursing drug handbook.)

Preoperative Medication	Action	Onset and Duration

7. What procedures were performed on Clarence Hughes before his surgery was begun? (*Hint:* Continue reviewing the Surgical Reports section in the chart.)

8. Clarence Hughes' surgery lasted _____.

9. What was tobramycin used for during this surgery?

10. What is in Clarence Hughes' history that makes it especially important for him to be diligent in using his incentive spirometer after surgery? (*Hint:* See the System Review section of the Surgical Reports.)

LESSON 21

Postoperative Care

Reading Assignment: Diet Therapy and Assisted Feeding (Chapter 27)
Care of the Surgical Patient (Chapter 37)
Providing Wound Care and Treating Pressure Ulcers
(Chapter 38)
Promoting Musculoskeletal Function (Chapter 39)

Patients: Clarence Hughes, Medical-Surgical Floor, Room 404
Piya Jordan, Medical-Surgical Floor, Room 403
Kathryn Doyle, Skilled Nursing Floor, Room 503

Objectives:

- Discuss necessary elements of the PACU report to the floor.
- Identify assessments necessary for a patient returning to the nursing unit from surgery.
- Prioritize care for the fresh postoperative patient.
- Assist with convalescence and recovery after surgery.

Exercise 1

 CD-ROM Activity—Postoperative Care After Knee Replacement

 30 minutes

- Sign in to work at Pacific View Regional Hospital on the Medical-Surgical Floor for Period of Care 1. (*Note:* If you are already in the virtual hospital from a previous exercise, click on **Leave the Floor** and then **Restart the Program** to get to the sign-in window.)
- From the Patient List, select Clarence Hughes (Room 404).
- Click on **Go to Nurses' Station** and then on **Chart**.
- Select the chart for **404** and click on **Physician's Orders**. Review the postoperative orders for Clarence Hughes.

1. What is the purpose of continuous passive motion by machine after joint replacement surgery? (*Hint:* See page 791 in your textbook.)

2. What would you do before placing Clarence Hughes' knee in the CPM machine?

3. What is the goal for angle of flexion for today, the second postoperative day? Would you set the machine for this goal degree when beginning the procedure for the day?

4. How would you determine how well Clarence Hughes is tolerating the CPM machine?

5. Clarence Hughes is to ambulate twice a day. He will initially use a walker to do this. You

    know that the walker height is appropriate for him if his elbows are bent _____ degrees when his hands are on the handgrips and he is standing upright.

6. When checking the walker for safety, you would check to see that the

    _____ on the legs are intact.

➤ • Click on **Return to Nurses' Station** and then click on **404**.

   • Inside the patient's room, click on **Patient Care** and then on **Chest**. From the list of assessment subcategories (the green boxes), choose **Respiratory** and perform a respiratory assessment.

7. Clarence Hughes is at high risk of respiratory complications because he is a smoker. Record your findings from his respiratory assessment below.

→ • Now click on **EPR** and **Login**. Choose **404** in the Patient box. Choose **Respiratory** from the Category drop-down menu. Document your assessment findings from above.

• Scroll back through the previous respiratory findings.

8. Has Clarence Hughes been using his incentive spirometer regularly?

9. Clarence Hughes is to use his incentive spirometer regularly. Check his orders and then decide which of the following teaching points you should go over with him. Mark your choices with an X. (*Hint:* See page 733 in your textbook.)

_____ a. Exhale through the nose.

_____ b. Inhale slowly and deeply.

_____ c. Hold the inhalation for 3 seconds.

_____ d. Use the spirometer for 20 breaths with each use.

_____ e. Make the ball rise to the marker with each inhalation.

_____ f. Breathe normally between each breath on the spirometer.

_____ g. Exhale into the spirometer forcefully.

_____ h. Use the spirometer ten times each hour while awake.

_____ i. Pucker lips when exhaling.

Exercise 2

 CD-ROM Activity—Care of the Fresh Postoperative Patient

 30 minutes

- Sign in to work at Pacific View Regional Hospital on the Medical-Surgical Floor for Period of Care 1. (*Note:* If you are already in the virtual hospital from a previous exercise, click on **Leave the Floor** and then **Restart the Program** to get to the sign-in window.)
- From the Patient List, select Piya Jordan (Room 403).
- Click on **Go to Nurses' Station**.
- Click on **Chart** and then on **403**. Select the tab for **Physician's Orders**. Review the postoperative orders.

1. After you receive a fresh postoperative patient and get report from the PACU nurse, what initial assessments would you make once the patient is settled in the unit?

2. What is the schedule for the frequent vital sign measurements for a patient who has just returned from the operating room?

3. Assume that Piya Jordan is a fresh postoperative patient. Match each action below with the tube or device to which it applies.

Action	**Tube or Device**
_____ Assess amount of output every hour for first 4 hours.	a. IV
_____ Keep tubing above the level of the container.	b. NG tube
_____ Check site every 4 hours.	c. Foley catheter
_____ Position prongs curving downward.	d. Oxygen cannula
_____ Check flow rate every hour.	e. Dressing
_____ Set to low intermittent suction.	
_____ Assess for bleeding every 2 hours.	

4. Piya Jordan needs to be repositioned every 2 hours. How can she be positioned after this surgery?

→ • Click on **Return to Nurses' Station** and then on **403**.
  • Click on **Patient Care** and then on **Abdomen**.

5. Piya Jordan had an exploratory laparotomy and right hemicolectomy. For this reason, an abdominal assessment is of high priority. Assess each aspect of the abdominal area and record the findings below and on the next page. (*Hint:* To perform this assessment, click on each of the subcategories in the green boxes, as well as on the **Equipment** button to the right of the green boxes.)

Integumentary

Musculoskeletal

Gastrointestinal

Equipment

→ •   Now click on **EPR** and on **Login**. Select **403** in the Patient box and document your findings from Piya Jordan's abdominal assessment. To do so, you will need to access the **Gastrointestinal** and the **Wounds and Drains** flow charts, using the Category drop-down menu.

6. What effect may Piya Jordan's age have on her wound healing? (*Hint:* See pages 757-759 in your textbook.)

7. Piya Jordan is presently in the _____ stage of wound healing, which lasts

about _____ days. (*Hint:* See page 755 in your textbook.)

8. Piya Jordan has a _____ wound drainage device. (*Hint:* See page 761 of your textbook.)

9. What must be done after emptying the suction system in order to reactivate it?

10. Because Piya Jordan has had abdominal surgery, getting her to cough adequately will be difficult. Explain how you would prepare and assist her with coughing.

 11. The physician has ordered sequential compression devices for Piya Jordan. What is the purpose of these devices? (*Hint:* See page 746 in your textbook.)

Exercise 3

 CD-ROM Activity—Surgical Recovery and Medication Administration

 30 minutes

Kathryn Doyle is in the Skilled Nursing Unit recovering from hip surgery.

- Sign in to work at Pacific View Regional Hospital on the Skilled Nursing Floor for Period of Care 1. (*Note:* If you are already in the virtual hospital from a previous exercise, click on **Leave the Floor** and then **Restart the Program** to get to the sign-in window.)
- From the Patient List, select Kathryn Doyle (Room 503).
- Click on **Get Report** and read the note.
- Click on **Go to Nurses' Station** and then on **503**. Read the **Initial Observation**.

1. Kathryn Doyle has dry mucous membranes, which could indicate _____.

→ • Click on **Take Vital Signs**.

2. Kathryn Doyle's current vital signs are:

BP _____ SpO$_2$ _____ T _____ HR _____ RR _____ Pain level _____

→ • Click on **Patient Care** and perform a focused assessment on Kathryn Doyle, particularly looking for potential surgical complications.

3. What abnormalities did you find on the respiratory assessment for Kathryn Doyle?

4. Her Homans' sign was _____, and there is no evidence of the vascular

   complication of _____.

5. Encouraging Kathryn Doyle to drink water will help alleviate her _____,

   which may bring down her _____.

 • Click on **MAR** and see what medications are scheduled for Kathryn Doyle at 0800.

6. Below, list the medications you are to administer to Kathryn Doyle. For each, provide the
   classification and its action or the reason for giving it.

Medication Order	Classification	Action/Reason for Administration

 • Click on **Medication Room** on the bottom of your screen and begin to prepare Kathryn
   Doyle's 0800 medications.
 • Click on **Unit Dosage** or on the unit dosage cart. Select drawer **503**.
 • Using the five rights and the five responsibilities, follow the onscreen steps to select the 0800
   medications for Kathryn Doyle. For each selection, click on **Put Medication on Tray**.

7. Were there any problems with the medications that were in the drawer as compared with the
   orders?

8. What should you do?

• When all of the 0800 medications are on the tray, click on **Close Drawer**. Next, click **Review Medications**, performing the second check for each dose ordered for 0800.

- Click **Return to Medication Room** and then **View Medication Room**.

- Click on **Preparation** or on the tray on the left side of your screen.

- For each medication, click **Prepare** and provide the information requested by the Preparation Wizard.

- When all medications have been prepared, click on **Finish** and then on **Return to Medication Room**.

- Click on **503** to return to the patient's room. Click on **Patient Care** and then on **Medication Administration**.

- Administer each medication by clicking the down arrow next to **Select**, choosing **Administer** and following the prompts.

- When you have finished the 0800 medication administration, click on **Leave the Floor** and then on **Look at Your Preceptor's Evaluation**. Click on **Medication Scorecard** to see how you did.

9. What three things should you have done before you rechecked and opened the medication unit dose packages?

LESSON 22

Patient Teaching

🕮 **Reading Assignment:** Patient Teaching (Chapter 9)

Patients: Patricia Newman, Medical-Surgical Floor, Room 406
Clarence Hughes, Medical-Surgical Floor, Room 404
Piya Jordan, Medical-Surgical Floor, Room 403

Objectives:

- Identify areas of knowledge deficit for patients.
- Recognize factors that may affect learning for individual patients.
- Determine the best methods for teaching specific content.
- Devise individualized teaching plans.

It is a rare patient that does not have a knowledge deficit in some area. Teaching is an integral part of patient care. Sometimes teaching is very informal and takes place during the bath; other times it is structured into a more formal teaching-learning session. Learning needs must be assessed, a plan devised, and teaching carried out—all while trying to fit required care of the patient into the time allotted.

It is important to send home written instructions and care guides to reinforce your teaching. If a home health nurse will be caring for the patient at home and continuing the teaching, communicate the teaching plan to that nurse when the patient is discharged.

Exercise 1

  CD-ROM Activity—Assessing Learning Needs

 30 minutes

Review the factors that affect learning on pages 114-115 of your textbook.

- Sign in to work at Pacific View Regional Hospital on the Medical-Surgical Floor for Period of Care 3. (*Note:* If you are already in the virtual hospital from a previous exercise, click on **Leave the Floor** and then **Restart the Program** to get to the sign-in window.)
- From the Patient List, select Patricia Newman (Room 406).
- Click on **Go to Nurses' Station**.
- Click on **Chart** and then on **406**.
- Click on the **Nursing Admission** tab.

1. What factors mentioned in the chart do you think may interfere with learning for Patricia Newman at this time? Mark your choices with an X.

_____ a. Pain

_____ b. Fatigue

_____ c. Fever

_____ d. Anxiety

_____ e. Decreased oxygenation

_____ f. Nausea

_____ g. Sedation

_____ h. Visitor

Review the Modes of Learning and Factors Affecting Learning on pages 113-115 in your textbook.

2. Based on your review of the Nursing Admission assessment, you determine that Patricia

Newman most likely learns best by _____. This means that

Patricia Newman is primarily a(n) _____ (auditory/visual/kinesthetic) learner.

3. What methods would you employ in carrying out Patricia Newman's teaching plan?

4. Fill in the following form, assessing factors that might affect Patricia Newman's learning.

Factors Affecting Learning—Patricia Newman

Primary language:

Memory is:

Vision is:

Barriers to learning:

Secondary language:

Hearing:

Literacy level:

---

 5. Did you discover any cultural factors that might affect Patricia Newman's willingness to learn or the way you should plan teaching for her? (*Hint:* See Cultural Values and Expectations in your textbook on page 114.)

6. A nursing diagnosis related to Patricia Newman's learning needs would be _____

_____.

 • Click on **Return to Nurses' Station** and then on **406**.
• Inside the patient's room, click on **Patient Care** and then on **Nurse-Client Interactions**.
• Select and view the video titled **1500: Discharge Planning**. (*Note:* Check the virtual clock to see whether enough time has elapsed. You can use the fast forward feature to advance the time by two-minute intervals if the video is not yet available. Then click on **Patient Care** and **Nurse-Client Interactions** to refresh the screen.)
• After viewing the video, click on **Chart** and then on **406**. Select the **Patient Education** tab and read the education plan.

7. What seems to be missing from this plan considering the video interaction you just viewed?

8. List the eight areas of education that need to be addressed for Patricia Newman. (*Hint:* Review the dietary consult.)

9. Match the level of priority to the correct teaching area.

Teaching Area	Level of Priority
_____ Disease condition	a. First priority
_____ Smoking cessation	b. Second priority
_____ Diet management	
_____ Activity	
_____ Medication compliance	
_____ Self-care	

10. Which of the following resources do you think would be helpful for your teaching plan? Mark your choices with an X.

_____ a. Dietitian's help in planning meals

_____ b. Pictures of each medication

_____ c. Video on correct use of MDI

_____ d. Information and printed materials on community smoking cessation programs

_____ e. Drug inserts on her medications

_____ f. A chart for progress with progressive ambulation

_____ g. Booklet on emphysema and its treatment

_____ h. Statistics on death from smoking

_____ i. Chart and schedule for medication administration

_____ j. Demonstration of effective coughing

_____ k. Examples of high-protein snacks

_____ l. Pamphlet on proper MDI use

Exercise 2

  CD-ROM Activity—Teaching Self-Injection

30 minutes

- Sign in to work at Pacific View Regional Hospital on the Medical-Surgical Floor for Period of Care 2. (*Note:* If you are already in the virtual hospital from a previous exercise, click on **Leave the Floor** and then **Restart the Program** to get to the sign-in window.)
- From the Patient List, select Clarence Hughes (Room 404).
- Click on **Chart** and then on **404**. Click on the tab for **Nursing Admission** and read the assessment, noting factors that are pertinent to Clarence Hughes' learning.

1. Clarence Hughes has indicated that his best learning methods are _____

   _____.

2. How does Clarence Hughes describe his short- and long-term memory?

3. What problem does he indicate he has that will have an impact on teaching-learning sessions?

4. What would you do to help with this problem?

5. What other factor needs to be considered in particular to Clarence Hughes when planning his teaching-learning sessions?

6. Clarence Hughes will need to continue his enoxaparin injections at home. Use the format below to devise a teaching plan for him. (*Hint:* See pages 115-117 in your textbook.)

Teaching Plan

Topic	Behavioral Objective	Evaluation Method

7. Considering Clarence Hughes' education needs and his current condition, you must realize

that his pain _____.

8. You should also include _____ in the teaching-learning sessions.

Exercise 3

 CD-ROM Activity—Factors Affecting Learning

15 minutes

- Sign in to work at Pacific View Regional Hospital on the Medical-Surgical Floor for Period of Care 1. (*Note:* If you are already in the virtual hospital from a previous exercise, click on **Leave the Floor** and then **Restart the Program** to get to the sign-in window.)
- From the Patient List, select Piya Jordan (Room 403).
- Click on **Go to Nurses' Station**.
- Click on **Chart** and then on **403**.
- Review the **Laboratory Reports** and the **Nursing Admission**.
- Click on **Physician's Notes** and review the notes.

1. Which of the following factors might interfere with Piya Jordan's ability to learn at the present time? Mark your choices with an X.

   _____ a. Fatigue

   _____ b. Lack of family support

   _____ c. NPO status

   _____ d. Electrolyte imbalance

   _____ e. Poor hearing

   _____ f. Pain

   _____ g. Nausea

   _____ h. Tubes and drains

   _____ i. Anemia

   _____ j. Fear

   _____ k. Confusion

   _____ l. Inadequate oxygenation

2. Piya Jordan's best methods of learning are _____ and

   _____.

3. What level of education does Piya Jordan have?

4. Piya Jordan was formerly employed as a _____.

5. How might her former occupation be useful now?

6. If Piya Jordan's tumor turns out to be adenocarcinoma of the colon, she will need chemotherapy. Can you count on her husband to support her during treatment?

7. What other support might be available to Piya Jordan?

8. What cultural factors should be taken into consideration when formulating a teaching plan for Piya Jordan?

LESSON 23

Nursing Care of the Elderly

Reading Assignment: Promoting Healthy Adaptation to Aging (Chapter 13)
Lifting, Moving, and Positioning Patients (Chapter 18)
Common Physical Care Problems of the Elderly (Chapter 40)

Patients: William Jefferson, Skilled Nursing Floor, Room 501
Kathryn Doyle, Skilled Nursing Floor, Room 503

Objectives:

- Identify interventions to assist the confused elderly patient.
- Discuss age-related physiologic changes that predispose older adults to problems.
- Examine factors related to polypharmacy.
- Incorporate fall prevention measures into daily care.

Older adults may be very healthy, or they may have a variety of medical and physical problems. Safety is always a primary concern, and fall prevention is incorporated into every nursing care plan for the elderly patient. Most older adults fear developing dementia. If dementia does occur, the burden on the patient's spouse or other close family members can result in significant physical and emotional strain. Elder abuse is a major concern and occurs far more frequently than most people realize. Loneliness, depression, and hopelessness are frequently found in the elderly patient who has multiple health problems. Thorough holistic assessment and care can make a difference in the lives of these patients.

Exercise 1

 CD-ROM Activity—The Patient with Dementia

 30 minutes

- Sign in to work at Pacific View Regional Hospital on the Skilled Nursing Floor for Period of Care 1. (*Note:* If you are already in the virtual hospital from a previous exercise, click on **Leave the Floor** and then **Restart the Program** to get to the sign-in window.)
- From the Patient List, select William Jefferson (Room 501).
- Click on **Get Report** and review. Then click on **Go to Nurses' Station**.
- Click on **501** to visit William Jefferson. Read the **Initial Observation**.
- Click on **Chart** and then on **501**. Open the **History and Physical** and review.

1. What are the four main diagnoses that you find in the beginning of the History and Physical?

2. As you read further, you discover that William Jefferson also suffers from the musculo-

   skeletal disorder _____.

3. William Jefferson was hospitalized because of _____ and

   _____.

4. Physiologic changes that occur with aging in the male and contribute to the occurrence of

   the above problems are _____ and

   _____.

➜ • Click on **Return to Room 501** and then click on **Patient Care**.
   • Click on **Nurse-Client Interactions**.
   • Select and view the video titled **0730: Intervention—Patient Safety** and then the next video
     titled **0740: The Confused Patient**. (*Note*: Check the virtual clock to see whether enough
     time has elapsed. You can use the fast forward feature to advance the time by two-minute
     intervals if the video is not yet available. Then click on **Patient Care** and **Nurse-Client
     Interactions** to refresh the screen.)

5. What is the situation in the first interaction?

6. How does the second interaction demonstrate William Jefferson's confusion? What technique does the nurse use to handle the situation?

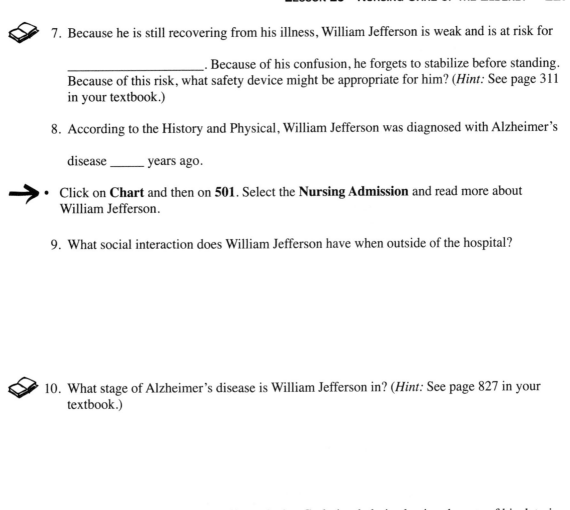

7. Because he is still recovering from his illness, William Jefferson is weak and is at risk for

_____. Because of his confusion, he forgets to stabilize before standing. Because of this risk, what safety device might be appropriate for him? (*Hint:* See page 311 in your textbook.)

8. According to the History and Physical, William Jefferson was diagnosed with Alzheimer's

disease _____ years ago.

→ • Click on **Chart** and then on **501**. Select the **Nursing Admission** and read more about William Jefferson.

9. What social interaction does William Jefferson have when outside of the hospital?

10. What stage of Alzheimer's disease is William Jefferson in? (*Hint:* See page 827 in your textbook.)

11. How do you think William Jefferson's dog Curly is a help in slowing the rate of his deterioration? (*Hint:* See page 835 in your textbook.)

Exercise 2

CD-ROM Activity—Physical Problems of the Elderly

45 minutes

Recall that William Jefferson was admitted with a urinary tract infection and sepsis. His diabetes and blood pressure were not controlled at the time of admission.

• Sign in to work at Pacific View Regional Hospital on the Skilled Nursing Floor for Period of Care 1. (*Note:* If you are already in the virtual hospital from a previous exercise, click on **Leave the Floor** and then **Restart the Program** to get to the sign-in window.)

• From the Patient List, select William Jefferson (Room 501).

• Click on **Get Report** and read the note.

• Click on **Go to Nurses' Station**.

1. How do decreased bladder tone and incomplete emptying predispose older adults to urinary tract infection? (*Hint:* See page 529 in your textbook.)

2. How does benign prostatic hypertrophy add to the problem of decreased bladder tone? (*Hint:* Read in your medical-surgical textbook about this disorder.)

3. Which of the following would you include in your teaching plan for William Jefferson and his wife in order to prevent recurrent cystitis? Mark your choices with an X.

_____ a. Increase fluid intake to 1800 mL per day.

_____ b. Empty the bladder every 2 hours.

_____ c. Drink cranberry juice daily.

_____ d. Take a Vitamin B_1 supplement.

_____ e. Increase fluid intake to 2500-3000 mL per day.

_____ f. Empty the bladder every hour.

_____ g. Avoid most citrus fruits and juice.

_____ h. Take a vitamin C supplement.

William Jefferson developed sepsis, which in this case was a systemic inflammatory response to the infection. Sepsis can be fatal. It is important that William Jefferson and his wife receive adequate teaching about prevention of future urinary tract infections. William Jefferson also has hypertension, diabetes, and osteoarthritis. He has several medications prescribed for his various conditions.

→ • Click on **MAR** and select tab **501** for William Jefferson's records.

4. Below, list the regularly scheduled medications prescribed for William Jefferson. For each medication, provide the action and explain why he is receiving it.

Medication Order	Action	Reason for Receiving

5. A person in William Jefferson's age range who has this many drugs prescribed is at risk for

_____. In this instance, William Jefferson needs most of these medications to control his various chronic conditions. When his infection has been adequately treated, he will no longer take the antibiotic.

 6. Why is taking multiple medications such a problem for an elderly person? (*Hint:* See page 818 in your textbook.)

7. Another factor that can contribute to drug toxicity in the elderly is _____.

8. The use of nonprescription drugs such as _____ or

_____ can alter drug elimination from the body.

- Click on **Return to Nurses' Station**. Now click on **Medication Room** and begin to prepare William Jefferson's 0800 medications.

- Click on **Unit Dosage** or on the unit dosage cart. Select drawer for **501** to see a list of the medications ordered for William Jefferson.

- Click on one of the drugs you need to administer at 0800.

- Compare the unit dosage label with the MAR order; then click **Put Medication on Tray**.

- Repeat the previous two steps for each 0800 medication.

- Now perform your second check by clicking on **Review Your Medications** and using the five rights.

- After verifying your medications, click on **Return to Medication Room**, then on **Close Drawer**, and then on **View Medication Room**.

- Click on **Preparation** in the upper left of your screen.

- Prepare each medication by clicking on the drug name and supplying any information requested by the Preparation Wizard.

- When all medications are properly prepared and verified, click on **Finish** and then on **Return to Medication Room**.

- Now click on **501**, **Patient Care**, and **Medication Administration**.

- Administer all of William Jefferson's 0800 medications using the five rights and following the prompts of the Administration Wizard.

- When finished, click on **Leave the Floor** and then on **Look at Your Preceptor's Evaluation**. Finally, select **Medication Scorecard** to see how you did.

9. Did you make any errors? If so, what were they? What would you do differently next time?

Exercise 3

 CD-ROM Activity—Fall Prevention

 15 minutes

- Sign in to work at Pacific View Regional Hospital on the Skilled Nursing Floor for Period of Care 1. (*Note:* If you are already in the virtual hospital from a previous exercise, click on **Leave the Floor** and then **Restart the Program** to get to the sign-in window.)
- From the Patient List, select Kathryn Doyle (Room 503).
- Click on **Get Report** and read the note.
- Click on **Go to Nurses' Station**.
- Now click on **Chart** and then on **503**. Click on the tab for **History and Physical**.

Kathryn Doyle is in the Skilled Nursing Unit for rehabilitation after the hip surgery.

1. What diagnoses are listed in the initial part of the History and Physical?

 • Click on **Return to Nurses' Station** and then on **503**.
- Click on **Clinical Alerts** and review the note.
- Click on **Patient Care** and then on **Nurse-Client Interactions**.
- Select and view the video titled **0730: Assessment—Biopsychosocial**. (*Note:* Check the virtual clock to see whether enough time has elapsed. You can use the fast forward feature to advance the time by two-minute intervals if the video is not yet available. Then click on **Patient Care** and **Nurse-Client Interactions** to refresh the screen.)

2. What two factors did you discover that might contribute to Kathryn Doyle's risk for a fall?

3. Her degree of fall risk would be considered _____ at this time.

• Click on **Kardex** and review the activity orders for Kathryn Doyle.

4. What does the Kardex say about Kathryn Doyle's activity orders?

5. When you assist Kathryn Doyle to get up from the bed to sit in the chair, you should take several actions in a particular sequence. Listed below are the actions you would need to take after positioning the chair next to the bed. Number these steps to show the order in which you would perform them. (*Hint:* See Chapter 18, page 263 in your textbook.)

_____ Assist her to sit.

_____ Put firm-soled slippers on her feet.

_____ Place a transfer belt around her waist.

_____ Ask her whether she is dizzy.

_____ Sit her up on the side of the bed.

_____ Allow a couple of minutes for her to dangle.

_____ Allow a couple of minutes for her blood pressure to stabilize.

_____ Help her to a standing position.

_____ Tell her what you are going to do.

_____ Lower the bed.

_____ Assist her to the chair, gripping the transfer belt.

→ • Click on **Return to Room 503** and then on **MAR**. Review Kathryn Doyle's MAR.

6. What medication is Kathryn Doyle receiving that could contribute to a fall? (*Hint:* To check her medications for side effects, consult the Drug Guide on the CD-ROM or use your pharmacology book or nursing drug handbook.)

Read about anemia in your medical-surgical textbook.

7. How can an anemic condition be a factor in a fall for an elderly person?

8. What devices would you recommend that the family install in Kathryn Doyle's bathroom at home to help prevent a future fall? (*Hint:* See Table 20-3 on page 310 in your textbook.)

LESSON 24

Psychosocial Care of the Elderly

 Reading Assignment: Promoting Healthy Adaptation to Aging (Chapter 13)
Common Psychosocial Care Problems of the Elderly
(Chapter 41)

Patients: Kathryn Doyle, Skilled Nursing Floor, Room 503
William Jefferson, Skilled Nursing Floor, Room 501
Clarence Hughes, Medical-Surgical Floor, Room 404

Objectives:

- Identify the various types of elder abuse.
- Determine factors that indicate an elderly person needs assistance.
- Assess developmental level factors in the elderly.
- Describe factors that might indicate depression in the elderly.

Exercise 1

CD-ROM Activity—Abuse, Depression, and Need for Assistance

30 minutes

- Sign in to work at Pacific View Regional Hospital on the Skilled Nursing Floor for Period of Care 3. (*Note:* If you are already in the virtual hospital from a previous exercise, click on **Leave the Floor** and then **Restart the Program** to get to the sign-in window.)
- From the Patient List, select Kathryn Doyle (Room 503).
- Click on **Go to Nurses' Station**.
- Click on **Chart** and then on **503**.
- Click on the **Nurse's Notes** tab and review the note regarding the incident with a family member.
- Click on **Consultations** and review.
- Next, click on **Nursing Admission** and review the data.

1. Depression is often overlooked in the elderly. The physician has ordered a psychiatric nurse consult for Kathryn Doyle. What information have you found in the chart that might contribute to depression for Kathryn Doyle?

→ • Click on **Return to Nurses' Station** and then on **503** to visit Kathryn Doyle.
   • Click on **Patient Care** and then on **Nurse-Client Interactions**.
   • Select and view the video titled **1505: Assessment—Elder Abuse**. (*Note*: Check the virtual clock to see whether enough time has elapsed. You can use the fast forward feature to advance the time by two-minute intervals if the video is not yet available. Then click on **Patient Care** and **Nurse-Client Interactions** to refresh the screen.)

 2. Which of the following assessment findings for depression does Kathryn Doyle exhibit? Mark your choices with an X. (*Hint*: Base your answers on the video interaction you just observed, as well as your review of the Nursing Admission, Consultations, and Nurse's Notes in the chart. Also see Table 41-8 on page 829 of your textbook.)

_____ a. Fatigue

_____ b. Envy/criticism of others

_____ c. Appetite changes

_____ d. "Not feeling good"

_____ e. Sleep pattern changes

_____ f. Poor outlook on life

_____ g. Headaches

_____ h. Memory impairment

_____ i. Feelings of worthlessness/helplessness

3. The psychiatric nurse specialist suggests that Kathryn Doyle be started on an

   _____ of the _____ type.

4. The primary responsibility of the nurse when a patient is started on this type of medication

   is to _____.

5. Kathryn Doyle has not been taken to the dentist to have her dentures fixed for a very long

   time, and she is having trouble eating. This could be considered as _____
   on the part of her son.

6. Kathryn Doyle's son will not let her cook, clean, or manage her own money. She has indicated that she feels useless. These actions on the part of her son might be considered what
   type of abuse?

7. After a parent dies, what signs would indicate that the surviving elderly spouse needs help
   and perhaps should not live alone? Mark your choices with an X. (*Hint:* See page 166 in
   your textbook.)

   _____ a. Frequent inability to find the right words

   _____ b. Forgetfulness

   _____ c. Withdrawal from others

   _____ d. Suspicion of others

   _____ e. Confusion about medications

   _____ f. Watching a lot of TV

   _____ g. Frequent falls

   _____ h. Social isolation

   _____ i. Unpaid bills

Exercise 2

  CD-ROM Activity—Therapeutic Communication and Medication

 30 minutes

- Sign in to work at Pacific View Regional Hospital on the Skilled Nursing Floor for Period of Care 3. (*Note:* If you are already in the virtual hospital from a previous exercise, click on **Leave the Floor** and then **Restart the Program** to get to the sign-in window.)
- From the Patient List, select William Jefferson (Room 501).
- Click on **Go to Nurses' Station**.
- Click on **MAR** and select tab **501**. Review William Jefferson's prescribed drugs.

1. The physician has prescribed _____ for William Jefferson's Alzheimer's disease.

- Click on **Return to Nurses' Station** and then click on the **Drug** icon in the lower left corner of the screen. Scroll to the drug you identified in question 1 and read about it.

2. Below is a list of the possible side effects of the drug that has been prescribed for William Jefferson's Alzheimer's disease. Match each side effect with its degree of frequency.

Side Effect	**Frequency of Side Effect**
_____ Syncope	a. Frequent
_____ Nausea	b. Occasional
_____ Insomnia	c. Rare
_____ Tremor	
_____ Diarrhea	
_____ Anorexia	
_____ Hypertension	
_____ Anxiety	
_____ Headache	
_____ Confusion	

3. Does William Jefferson have other problems that this drug could exacerbate? If so, explain.

4. What would you teach William Jefferson and his wife about this drug?

 • Click on **Return to Nurses' Station**.
- Click on **501** to visit William Jefferson.
- Click on **Patient Care** and perform a neurologic and mental status assessment by clicking first on **Head & Neck** and then on each of the subcategories in the green boxes.
- After you have finished the assessment, click on **Nurse-Client Interactions**.
- Select and view the video titled **1525: Living with Alzheimer's**. (*Note*: Check the virtual clock to see whether enough time has elapsed. You can use the fast forward feature to advance the time by two-minute intervals if the video is not yet available. Then click on **Patient Care** and **Nurse-Client Interactions** to refresh the screen.)

5. What is the first question the student nurse asks after sitting down?

 6. The question you identified above is an example of the therapeutic communication technique _____. (*Hint:* See pages 102-104 in your textbook.)

7. William Jefferson says that when he can't remember, it makes him feel stupid. What does the student nurse say in response to this? What therapeutic technique is she using here?

8. What is the primary goal of psychosocial interventions for the confused or disoriented elder? (*Hint:* See page 625 in your textbook.)

9. What are the other principles of care for the cognitively impaired elder? (*Hint:* See Table 41-3 on page 825 in your textbook.)

Exercise 3

 CD-ROM Activity—Developmental Tasks and Health Promotion

 30 minutes

- Sign in to work at Pacific View Regional Hospital on the Medical-Surgical Floor for Period of Care 1. (*Note:* If you are already in the virtual hospital from a previous exercise, click on **Leave the Floor** and then **Restart the Program** to get to the sign-in window.)
- From the Patient List, select Clarence Hughes (Room 404).
- Click on **Go to Nurses' Station**.
- Click on **Chart** and then on **404**.
- Click on the tab for **Nursing Admission** and review the data.

   1. Clarence Hughes is _____ years old. He is in Erikson's stage of

      _____ and appears to be in _____.

 2. What information tells you that Clarence Hughes is in the positive side of this developmental phase? (*Hint:* See Table 11-1 on page 132 in your textbook. Use critical thinking for this question.)

   3. In contrast to Clarence Hughes, Kathryn Doyle is in the _____ phase of this developmental level. (*Hint:* Base your answer on what you learned about Kathryn Doyle in Exercise 1 of this lesson.)

4. What data from Exercise 1 support your answer to question 3?

5. Considering the data you have collected on Clarence Hughes, match the following actions with the best description in the right column.

Actions	**How It Applies**
_____ Obtains a flu shot each year	a. Health promoting
_____ Wears a seat belt when in the car	b. Risk to good health
_____ Obtains a prostate exam	c. Not performed by him
_____ Smokes cigarettes	
_____ Drinks alcohol occasionally	
_____ Watches TV most of the time	
_____ Performs testicular self-exams	
_____ Keeps weight within a normal range	
_____ Takes a vitamin-mineral supplement daily	
_____ Uses medications for glaucoma regularly	

 6. After his rehabilitation period, what health promotion behaviors would you recommend to Clarence Hughes? (*Hint:* See Chapter 13 in your textbook.)

7. What health promotion behaviors would you recommend for Kathryn Doyle? (*Hint:* Review your findings in Exercise 1 of this lesson. If necessary, go to the Skilled Nursing Floor and review the Nursing Admission and Consultations in her chart—Room 503.)

Notes:

Notes:

Notes: